I'm Pregnant
& I Have a Cold

Are Over-the-Counter
Drugs Safe to Use?

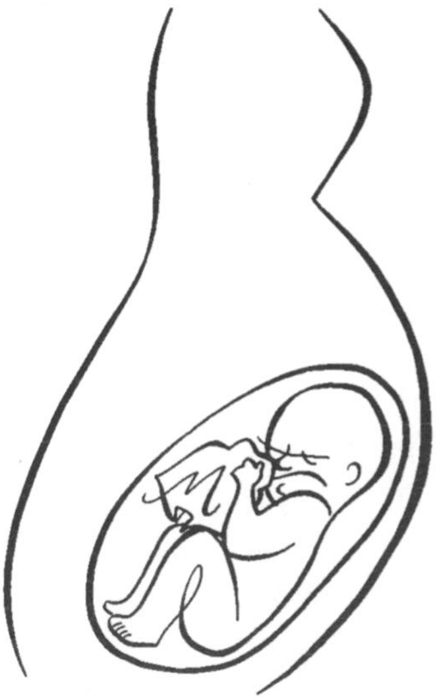

Craig V. Towers, M.D., F.A.C.O.G.

Acknowledgements:

Copy Editor:	Vera J. Belich
Book Design:	Barbara P. Infranca
Cover Illustration:	Kathryn Adams
Book Illustrations:	Kathryn Adams Denise Thompson

A special thanks to Ed Broder for his endless generosity.

Published by:
RBC Press, Inc., Huntington Beach, California

Please direct all correspondence and book orders to:

RBC Press, Inc.
9121 Atlanta Ave., Box 640, Huntington Beach, CA 92646
www.rbcpress.com (877) 935-5222

Library of Congress Catalog Card Number
99-075802

ISBN Number
0-9652016-6-X Soft Cover
0-9652016-7-8 Hard Cover

Printed in the United States of America by
B & L Lithograph
Huntington Beach, California

This book is dedicated to my wife Kelly, and my three wonderful children Rachel, Brian, and Chelsea. Without any question, they supported my decision to write this book which had been a dream of mine for several years. Their faith in me helped to make my dream become a reality.

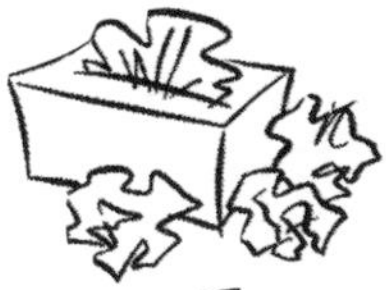

Table of Contents

Introduction

This is the first book in a series of three or four books that will discuss the use of over-the-counter (OTC) drugs in pregnancy. For more than ten years I have had an intense interest in over-the-counter drugs and their possible effects on pregnant women. Although some of these medications have been around for years, many have never been thoroughly studied to determine how safe they may be for use during pregnancy. Therefore, after researching this topic in great detail, I decided to put my thoughts and findings down on paper.

As this project evolved and research was compiled, it became clear that this topic was too big to be covered in one book. If every over-the-counter drug were placed in one book, it would be so enormous that many individuals might be scared off by the size alone. In addition, I wanted to make this information available to all pregnant women. Let's face it, the larger the book, the more expensive it becomes. Therefore, I decided to take the topic of OTC drugs and break it down into a few books, each covering a major type of ailment. By doing this, the cost would be minimized and pregnant women could tailor their selections to their specific needs.

In this first book alone, over 50 active ingredients are discussed in detail. These drugs (alone or in combination with others) make up thousands of products that are available for sale to the public.

Some people believe that using drugs during pregnancy should never happen. Is this belief correct? For some pregnant women the answer is yes! For others, however, using a medication may be helpful. This is because every pregnant woman is different. Let me give you an example.

Some women can develop a problem very early in pregnancy where their cervix dilates or opens up without contractions. For treatment, they are put to bed and instructed to stay off their feet. These women must still have bowel movements, but is it prudent for them to strain in order to pass stool? The answer is no, because straining could cause the cervix to open even more or make the membranes (bag of water) break. Therefore, giving these women a stool softener is often helpful.

Furthermore, everybody has to deal with stress, and how stress is handled varies from person to person. One woman may be able to tolerate a tremendous amount of stress with few problems, whereas another woman may not tolerate it at all. Stress is known to release natural chemicals in our bodies that can affect us in many ways. Stress may lead to high blood pressure, stomach problems, headaches, and ulcers, to name a few.

Trying to determine what stress can do during a pregnancy is difficult because there is no reliable scientific way to measure levels of stress. There is one study which took a group of women who had two pregnancies—one pregnancy occurred while the women were in training to become doctors and the other pregnancy occurred after their training was complete. There were less problems and complications in the pregnancies that occurred after the training was completed, despite the fact that the women were now older. Usually, the older a woman becomes, the chance for complications will either stay the same or increase, especially for high blood pressure, diabetes, and other medical problems. Therefore, putting stress aside, the expected complication rate would be the same or higher during the second pregnancy (when the women were older). The fact that the first pregnancy had the higher complication rate may reflect the effect of stress experienced during their medical training.

Some individuals when infected with a cold or flu virus never really become very sick. On the other hand, some people always have a terrible time. Being infected with a cold or flu virus is a stress to the body. Therefore, treating the symptoms of a severe cold for some women may decrease stress and be helpful.

Unfortunately, no one can ever tell you—the pregnant mom—that using an over-the-counter medication is completely safe, because every pregnancy is unique. When it comes to taking drugs during pregnancy, the decision to use a medicine or not must be made by you with your healthcare provider and with your partner. At this point, you may be thinking, "Then what good is this book?" The purpose of this book is to inform pregnant women what cold remedies and related drugs can and cannot do and to help guide women and their healthcare providers in choosing the best over-the-counter drug for a specific condition. This book goes beyond describing individual medications. It provides women with important information about the overall topic of drugs in pregnancy including what effects they may have besides birth defects and how drug safety is determined.

This book is presented in two parts. Part One contains important information that all pregnant women should know. Part Two provides specific details about cold and flu virus infections and discusses cold remedy medications and related drugs that can be used to treat certain symptoms.

If the information within these pages becomes helpful to even one pregnant woman then I will consider the book a success. We must remember that our babies and our children are the future of this world, and anything that we can do to make their chances better will be good for the entire human race. As an obstetrician and perinatologist (a physician who specializes in high-risk pregnancies), *I have been blessed* that women have allowed me the privilege to care for them during their pregnancies and to participate in the glorious event of the births of their children. Nothing in life could be more spectacular!

I.

Part I.

What The

Well-Informed

Mother-To-Be

Should Know.

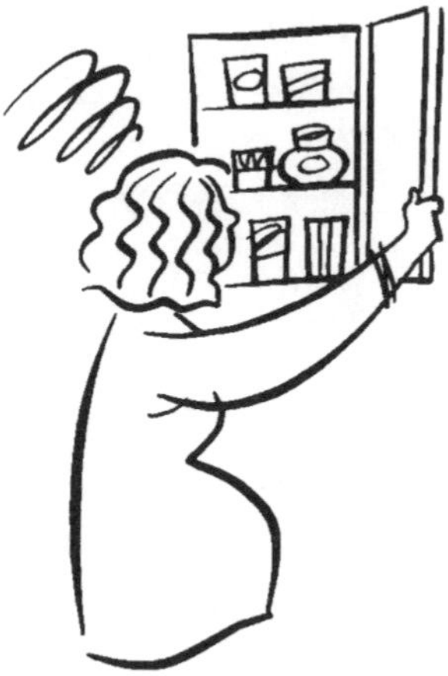

1. What Should I Know About Over-The-Counter Medications?

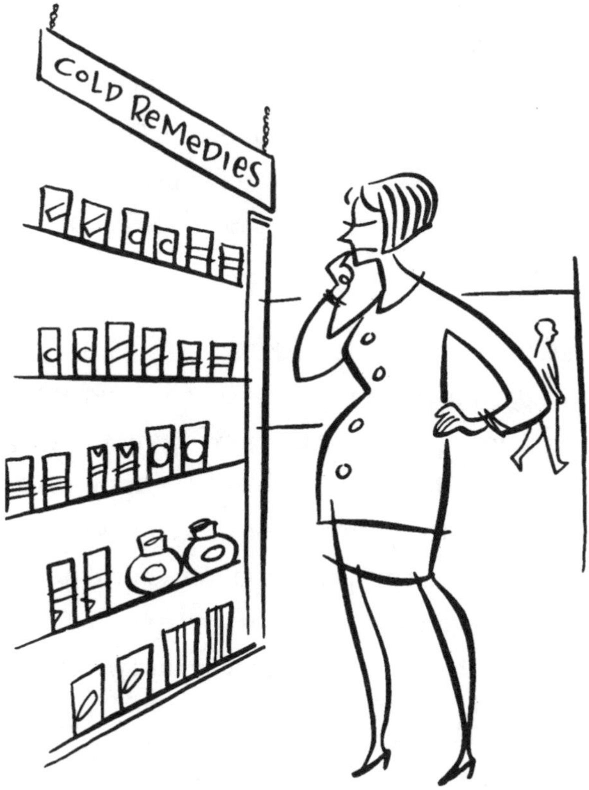

Over-the-counter medications can be purchased without a prescription, and at the present time, several hundred active ingredients comprise the drugs sold on the market. The first few chapters of this book will provide some background information on drugs in general and their possible effects on a pregnancy. The remaining chapters will discuss the specific drugs. What follows below are little pieces of information that are important for all pregnant women (and even for some who are not pregnant) to know.

Generally Speaking

Many different medical drugs are available on the market today. Some of these can only be obtained from a pharmacy by means of a prescription from your doctor. Other medicines can be bought without a prescription and are often called over-the-counter (OTC) medications. They may also be called non-prescription drugs.

Not A Cure

The definition of an over-the-counter drug in this book is the **actual active chemical** that may (or may not) do something to you when it is used or taken. This is important to understand because often an over-the-counter medication may contain more than one active drug. You should also know that these medicines are **not a cure** for the problem that you may have developed; they only try to make the symptoms less severe so you feel better.

The Name Game

The names on the packages of medications that you can buy over-the-counter are called **brand names** or **trade names**. For example, aspirin is an over-the-counter drug and is one of the medications that can be taken for pain. Aspirin, however, is marketed by several different drug companies and each gives it their own trade name (Ascriptin, Bufferin, Ecotrin, and Excedrin are examples). Therefore, as you read this book, keep in mind that the drugs listed are NOT the names on the bottles and boxes that stare back at you from the shelf. The drugs in this book are the actual active ingredients.

The reason this book was written in this fashion is because the active ingredients, the combination of the ingredients, and/or the amount of an active drug may change over time in a particular OTC medication because of modifications or potential improvements (or marketing considerations) designed by the drug company. Furthermore, many different trade names may exist worldwide for the same drug (as briefly shown in the aspirin example above) and to list them all would be next to impossible (over 200,000 are sold in the United States alone). Therefore, individual active ingredients are discussed in this book so the information can be applied to any OTC medication you might purchase now or in the future.

After reading the above paragraph, you probably have come to the conclusion that you will have to exert some effort and caution in buying an OTC medication. This is true because you will have to pick the item up off the shelf and read the list of ingredients that are contained in a particular product (the fine print often requires a magnifying glass). If you cannot read the label, please have someone read it to you to make sure that what is being bought and/or taken is the intended medication.

Quick Change Artist

Not to sound like a broken record, but here's an actual example of how one manufacturer of a particular OTC drug product completely changed the active ingredient but did not change the brand name (trade name). There is an over-the-counter medication that is used for treating leg pain (especially leg pain that happens at night when a person is trying to go to sleep). At one time, the active ingredient was **quinine** (KWY-nine). Following the U.S. Food and Drug Administration's review of this ingredient, quinine was no longer approved for use as an over-the-counter medication. However, the brand name drug can still be purchased for treating leg pain. Now the active ingredients are a combination of acetaminophen (a common pain medication) and diphenhydramine (an antihistamine). As brand names become established with the public, people become familiar and comfortable with the names, and they consider them to be safe and effective. They may not realize that the contents were completely changed. Therefore, the brand names may remain the same, but the active ingredients can be altered. By the way, quinine IS NOT A SAFE DRUG to take during pregnancy and has been known to cause miscarriages and stillbirths. BE ON THE ALERT! Quinine can still be found over-the-counter in **natural remedies** (homeopathic medications) for treating leg cramps. DO NOT USE these products while pregnant.

Not only should you take note of the **active** ingredients, you should also consider the **inactive** ingredients of any OTC drug that you might take. What is considered inactive may surprise you.

A Drug By Any Other Name

In my research, I discovered that about one-half to three-fourths of the population will buy and use an OTC medication without consulting a physician or someone in the healthcare profession. Since a pregnant woman must also consider the baby, she should learn as much as possible about OTC medications that could potentially cause harm.

Many people (pregnant women included) do not think that **over-the-counter medications are real drugs** or they may forget they are drugs. An example of this was shown in a report about a group of individuals who were seen at a medical clinic. In each original medical history obtained, the patient was asked whether he or she had taken any medications recently. When the examination was completed, the patients were seen by a dietician who reviewed their eating habits and also reviewed a list of several common over-the-counter drugs. The patients were asked if they had recently used any of the listed OTC products. Of those who answered yes, three out of four had answered no in the original history and physical form.

Evidently, many people forget that over-the-counter drugs ARE drugs, or they feel that these products must be safe or they wouldn't be available over-the-counter. Please remember that while most OTC drugs are relatively safe, some have the potential to be dangerous. If you happen to take an over-the-counter medication and then later find out you are pregnant, be sure to discuss this with your healthcare provider. If you are one of these individuals, you are not alone and you are not a bad person. However, what you took, the amount taken, and when it was used may be important information to include in your prenatal records.

More Is Not Better

Many of you know that some over-the-counter products also come as prescription drugs. The basic difference between the OTC pill and the prescription pill is the strength. The prescription pill usually contains more milligrams of the active ingredient in a given dose. However, increasing the amount of the over-the-counter medication for the purpose of equaling a prescription dose **should not be done**. Please follow the directions on the label of any over-the-counter medication you purchase and never take more than the recommended dose. If you want to increase the dosage, you must talk with your healthcare provider first, especially if you are pregnant!

The above paragraph is very, very important. It is not true that if a little helps then more must be better. Not following directions can lead to serious problems. Below is a real-life example.

An Example Of Overuse

Some women can develop problems during their pregnancy or they may have a medical illness like diabetes where the baby could be at risk. What is often done in complicated pregnancies is a procedure called **fetal monitoring**. In fetal monitoring, a belt is placed around the pregnant mother's abdomen or belly and positioned to lie across the uterus. Attached to this belt is a small device that can pick up the baby's heartbeat. This device sends information to a machine that will print out the recorded baby's heartbeats onto a continuous flowing strip of paper. This type of recording may also be used when you are in labor. When fetal monitoring is performed before a woman goes into labor, it is often called a non-stress test, a contraction stress test, or just plain fetal monitoring.

One of my patients had been having fetal monitoring twice a week to make sure that her baby was okay. On one particular visit, the baby's heartbeat was faster than normal. (By the way, the normal range for the heartbeat of most babies is 120 to 160 beats per minute.) Nothing else was wrong with the fetal monitoring evaluation except for the faster heart rate of 170 to 180 beats per minute. The mother-to-be told me that she had developed a cold a few days before this visit and had taken an over-the-counter cold remedy. In talking with her further, she stated that the normal dose and the normal schedule for taking the medication had not worked so she was using twice (or double) the recommended dosage, and she was taking it twice as often (instead of four times a day she was taking it up to eight times a day). The baby was active and the patient had no other complaints except for the cold symptoms. She stated that she did not have a fever with the cold and, at the time of her visit for the fetal monitoring, her temperature was normal. She was told to stop taking the medication and repeat the fetal monitoring in a few hours. When she did this, the baby's heart rate had returned to the normal range and the fetal monitor strip showed no signs of any problem. She eventually delivered a normal, healthy child a few weeks later. Examples of the fetal monitor tracings are seen in figure 1.

Some ingredients found in OTC medications can increase a person's heart rate. In the above case, the overuse of the drug allowed for more of it to cross over to the baby thereby increasing its heart rate. Remember, when using over-the-counter medications, **more is not better, more can cause problems for you, and more can harm your baby**!

Figure 1: Examples of fetal monitoring tracings.

Fast: *Fetal monitor tracing when the medication was used in excess, causing the baby's heart beat baseline to range from 180-190. The normal range should be 120-160 beats per minute.*

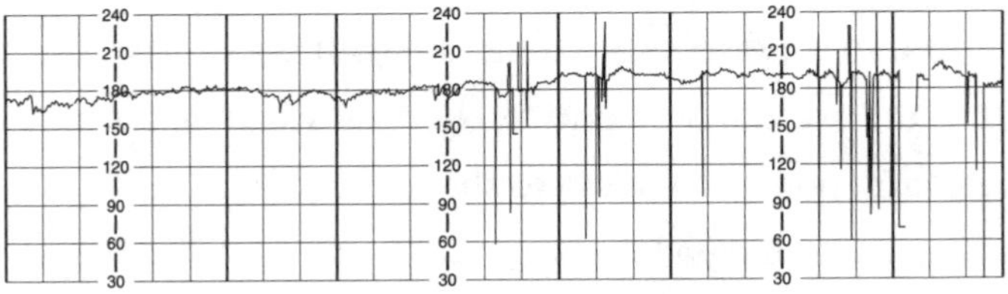

Monitor for uterine contractions, two contractions seen at the arrows.

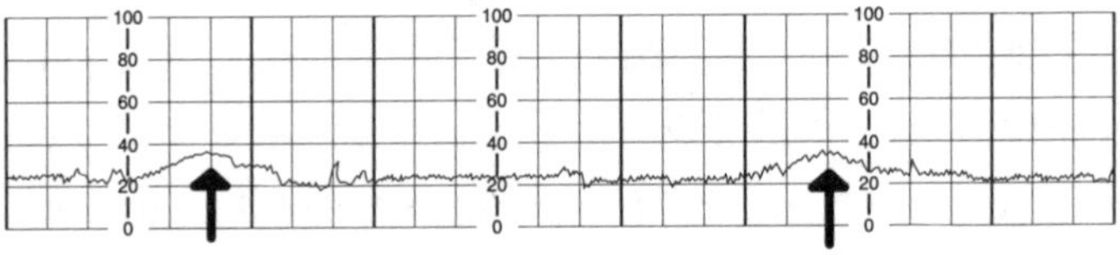

Normal: *Several hours after the drug was discontinued, the baby's heart beat baseline is now 140 beats per minute which is in the normal range.*

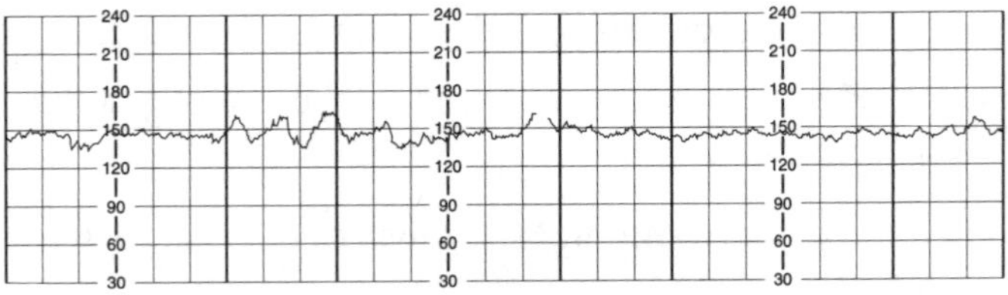

Monitor for uterine contractions, no contractions seen.

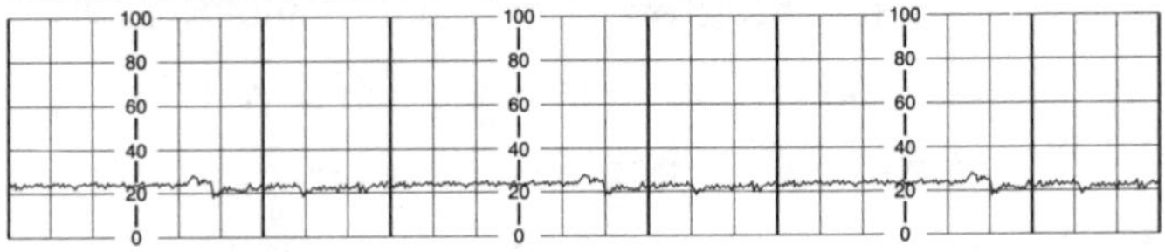

Playing Doubles

Because OTC products often contain more than one active ingredient, you should **be careful not to double up on medications**. Several different pain medications can be purchased over-the-counter. However, some of the same ingredients may also be found in OTC cold remedies. Therefore, if a person takes an aspirin along with a cold remedy (that also contains aspirin), in effect, the person is doubling the dose of aspirin. Another example is combining a hemorrhoid cream (that contains a decongestant-type drug) with an OTC cold remedy that has a decongestant or a nighttime sleep-aid (that is an antihistamine-type drug) with an allergy treatment also consisting of an antihistamine. The message here is to read the labels, especially if you plan on using more than one drug at a time, and make sure that no ingredients are duplicated.

The Opposite Of Wine

Many red wines will improve with age. Drugs, however, do not. This is why they all have expiration dates listed somewhere on the package. Any time a medication is used, you should always check the expiration date. Old medications do not turn into poison; however, they can become ineffective. Thus, they may not perform the desired function. In addition, as medicines become older, the color and taste can also change.

It is often said that old drugs may be harmful. This statement is basically true; however, the harm is not from the drug itself but rather from its lack of function. If a person is using an expired high blood pressure medication, he or she may not realize their blood pressure could still be high because the drug may no longer be effective.

Aspirin is one medication that may become more acidic (acid-like) over time and could cause more irritation to the stomach lining. Otherwise, most expired OTC products just lose their usefulness. Many people have medicine cabinets that are full of old medicine bottles (many of which have expired). The point of this discussion is to read the labels for expiration dates (as well as ingredients) and to discard all expired medications.

A Name For All Reasons

The term healthcare provider is used throughout this book because not all pregnant women are seen by obstetricians. Pregnant women may receive their prenatal care from a family practitioner, a nurse midwife, an outside clinic which is run by nurse practitioners, or other people who work in the healthcare industry. Therefore, this term is applied to whomever you may see for prenatal care (and you definitely should have prenatal care).

Considering Birth Defects

About 3.5 million to 4 million women give birth in the United States each year. Unfortunately, a baseline risk exists for having a child with a birth defect, and about two percent of all babies delivered in any given year will have a major birth defect (approximately 80,000). **Please don't let this number scare you** because statistics should always be looked at forwards and backwards. Thus out of 4,000,000 babies delivered, 3,920,000 **will not** have a major birth defect. Furthermore, if one were to add in all types of minor birth defects, a total of four to seven percent of all the babies delivered each year could have some type of defect (approximately 150,000 to 300,000). This also means that 3,700,000 to 3,850,000 babies will not have any birth defects whatsoever. An important issue to understand is that **only about five percent of all birth defects are attributed to drugs**. The majority of birth defects are either caused by genetic problems or at least are influenced by genetics.

The Baseline Risk

It should be noted at this point that if one were to study a group of pregnant women who took a specific drug during their pregnancy, at least two to four percent of them would deliver babies with birth defects unrelated to the drug. To explain this further, if we studied 100 pregnant women who were healthy and never took a single drug while pregnant, two to four of the babies delivered would still have some type of birth defect (and 96 to 98 would not have a birth defect). If a similar group of women took a drug during their pregnancy, at least two to four would have a child with a birth defect just like the group of women who took no medication during the pregnancy. The point is two to four babies with a birth defect (out of every 100 babies) is the **baseline risk** for birth defects.

In order to claim that a drug has a potential for causing birth defects, a study would have to show an increase in the baseline rate (greater than two to four percent), and the increase would have to be statistically significant, or it would have to be associated with an unusually high number of cases with a specific type of birth defect. Therefore, **every study** involving women who took a medication while pregnant **will show** that some babies had a birth defect because there is always a baseline risk. To repeat this, in order to claim that a drug causes birth defects, there must be a significant increase in the number seen over the baseline risk or there must be a clear indication of an increase in a specific type of birth defect.

Nothing To Fear But Fear

If any book covers the topic of pregnancy, it most likely would discuss potential problems that could develop. Some women may try to avoid learning about such problems because they might get "what if?" worries. If you are one of these individuals, you need to understand that information about potential problems contained in this book is solely intended to help you, not to frighten you. What you should know is that the overwhelming majority of pregnant women carry to full term and deliver healthy babies.

Allergies On A Scale Of Minor To Life-Threatening

Although an adverse reaction to any substance can be considered an allergy, this discussion specifically refers to **drug allergies**. Some allergies may cause a person to experience minor irritations such as a rash, hives, itching, or watery eyes. A drug allergy can also (in rare cases) be life-threatening and may involve tongue and throat swelling and severe shortness of breath (choking). This type of severe reaction is called anaphylaxis (AN-uh-fuh-LAK-sis).

If a person takes a drug and develops nausea and/or vomiting, this response is most likely an **intolerance** to the medication and not really an allergy. This may seem like I'm splitting hairs, but knowing the difference between an allergy, anaphylaxis, and intolerance may be very useful to you someday. Your healthcare provider will probably list your intolerance-type reaction as an allergy in your medical records (just as long as he or she doesn't refer to you as that intolerant patient).

Another important issue to discuss regarding allergies is **which ingredient** caused the reaction. Remember, OTC medications consist of the active ingredients along with several other chemicals. These might include caffeine, sugar substitutes, preservatives, lubricants, gels, flavorings, and colorings, to name a few. Therefore, an allergic reaction may not have been caused by one of the active ingredients but rather some other substance found in the medication. If you experience an allergic reaction to a drug, remember that any one of the chemicals found in the product could be the culprit.

No Information Overload

When you read about individual drugs in this book, the most common information is usually discussed. There is no way to fully describe everything that **might** happen when a drug is used, especially since some individuals experience very unusual reactions. In addition, attempting to list every possible problem that might occur after taking a specific drug would result in so much information that most people would just stop reading.

Do You Call This Penmanship?

Because some drugs have very similar names, when looking at medications taken off the shelf, you should always read the label on the package to be absolutely sure it's what you want. This is also very important when you pick up a prescription drug from a pharmacy.

Most doctors have illegible handwriting and oftentimes the pharmacist must read something that looks like hieroglyphics or some awful scribble. There could be a prenatal vitamin that has a trade name which is only one or two letters different than the trade name for a high blood pressure medication. Although pharmacists are trained to interpret medical "scribbles," let's say one busy afternoon the prescription is misread by the pharmacist and he or she fills the bottle with a high blood pressure medication. A normal healthy pregnant woman who thinks she is taking a prenatal vitamin could have serious problems if she uses the high blood pressure medication.

Remember, even when you pick up a prescription drug from the pharmacist, it is very important that you find out what the drug is for and be sure that it matches your understanding as to why your doctor gave you the prescription in the first place. This practice should also be extended to over-the-counter medications, especially if one is recommended to you by someone who uses the trade name. You **must** read the label carefully and be sure that the drug you are about to buy is the one you were intending to purchase.

For Informational Purposes Only

PLEASE don't take the information about the individual drugs discussed in this book as though they are recommended by me for use during a pregnancy. No one can ever know the complete story on the safety of a drug in a given pregnancy because everyone is unique and some people may have a different response to the drug when compared to another person. If you alone, or if you and your significant other, or if you and your healthcare provider decide that using one of the OTC medications is appropriate during your pregnancy, this book will hopefully guide you to the safest choice. In some cases, I might tell you which one my wife and I would choose, but that would be as far as this book could go. This book is NOT intended to replace the advice of your healthcare provider.

Sources

Information about the drugs discussed in this book was collected from several sources. The most prominent were the U.S. Food and Drug Administration (FDA), the Physicians' Desk Reference (PDR), and literature searches through medical libraries and computer programs (please see the bibliography). Every attempt was made to include all of the over-the counter drugs (for the listed categories) in the United States that can be used for treating certain symptoms. However, if you come across a drug that is not found in this book, you should talk with your healthcare provider to obtain further information.

Where Was The Drug Purchased?

Another very important piece of information is that this book describes the available over-the-counter drugs that can be bought in the United States. The active ingredients that may be found in drugs from other countries may very well be different. Therefore, if you are pregnant and you have an over-the-counter medication that was bought outside of the United States (assuming U.S. Customs didn't confiscate it), I recommend that you talk with your healthcare provider before you use it.

Drug Absorption

As you read further, you will see the word **absorb** used frequently. When talking about drugs in pregnancy, absorb means how much of the drug is pulled into the bloodstream.

Drugs or medicines can be absorbed into the bloodstream from the stomach or intestines if the drug is taken orally as a pill or liquid. Drugs or medicines can also be absorbed from the lining of the nose, mouth, rectum, vagina, and even from the eyes. The amount that is absorbed will differ from person to person, and the amount that is absorbed from the stomach may be different than the amount absorbed from the nose.

Another important fact to understand is that when a drug is absorbed into the body, that drug goes everywhere. For example, your doctor gives you a prescription for an antibiotic to heal a bladder infection. When you take the antibiotic, it will be absorbed into the bloodstream and will go to the bladder to fight the infection. The antibiotic, however, will also go through the rest of the body, including the heart, brain, lungs, and uterus. If you are pregnant, that antibiotic will also go by the placenta inside the uterus and may cross over to the baby. Therefore, if a substance is used during a pregnancy and is absorbed into the bloodstream, it has the potential of affecting the baby.

Words To Know

When reading about the medications, you may see words such as **onset, duration,** and **half-life**. The onset tells you how quickly you might see the effect of the drug after it is taken. The duration tells you roughly how long the effect may last, and the half-life tells you how long it takes for the body to remove one-half of the drug from the bloodstream.

You will also come across such words as **conception, embryo**, and **fetus.** Conception means that the egg from the woman and the sperm from the man have joined together to potentially produce another human being. The word embryo is the name that is given to the very early stages of the baby when it only consists of a group of cells. Later, when it becomes more recognizable as a baby, it is called a fetus.

Finally

If you are using a prescription drug, remember to talk with your healthcare provider before you take any over-the-counter medicine to be sure there is no overlap or conflict between the two drugs. If you have any medical problems such as high blood pressure, heart disease, or diabetes, you should definitely talk with your doctor before using any over-the-counter drug. Remember, **OTC medications are drugs**, and any drug taken during a pregnancy may also affect the baby you are carrying.

2. How Can Medicines Affect My Pregnancy?

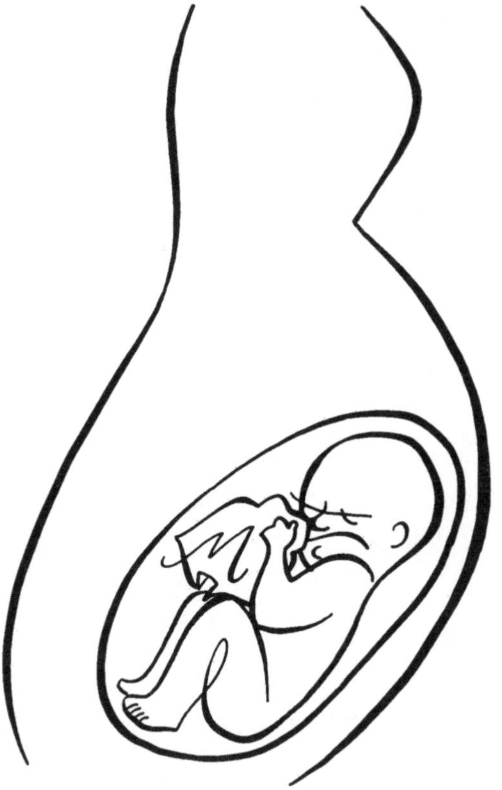

What are the concerns in taking medications while pregnant? Most pregnant couples (for those dads who are also interested) when asked this question wonder if their babies will be normal. Although drugs or medications can affect a pregnancy in several different ways, the fact is, very few have been proven to cause birth defects. Genetic factors are probably the most common cause for the majority of babies born with imperfections. By the way, some other words used for birth defect are birth anomalies, congenital defects, or congenital anomalies.

It is very easy to read several pages about what could go wrong in a pregnancy, but I want you to know that the overwhelming majority of pregnant women do well and deliver normal healthy babies. Therefore, even though the next several pages of this chapter talk about the different ways a drug **might** affect a pregnancy, remember that these issues are in the minority, NOT the majority. Some of the ways a medication could affect a pregnancy are as follows:

1. Drugs might cause birth defects.
2. Drugs might cause one of the baby's organs to not function properly leading to damage somewhere else.
3. Drugs might lead to problems that show up later in life.
4. Drugs might interfere with the function of the placenta (or afterbirth).
5. Drugs might interfere with labor.
6. Drugs might interfere with how the baby adapts to just being born.

1. Drugs might cause birth defects.

Lets start with the issue of birth defects because this is the biggest concern and raises the most questions. If a drug causes a birth defect, it is called a **teratogen** (tuh-RAT-tuh-jen), and the potential for a drug to cause birth defects is called its teratogenic (tuh-RAT-tuh-JEN-ic) potential, literally meaning monster forming. As stated earlier, very few drugs have been proven to cause birth defects. To begin with, if a drug is going to cause a birth anomaly, it has to be absorbed into the woman's bloodstream when she is pregnant.

Drugs Need To Be Absorbed!

The word absorb was defined in Chapter 1. However, to review, when we discuss drug absorption, we are talking about medicines that are taken either by mouth, placed in the rectum or vagina, placed in the nose or eye, or rubbed onto the skin. If a drug is given by injection, by definition, it will be picked up by the body and will travel through the bloodstream. However, medicines that are swallowed, or placed inside the rectum, vagina, nose, or eye, or rubbed onto the skin in the form of a cream or ointment may or may not be absorbed into the bloodstream. This is important to understand because if the drug is not absorbed into the bloodstream, or if only a little is absorbed, then the baby will be exposed to very little (if any) of the drug while it is in the mother's womb.

To simplify this, the baby is in its own little world inside the uterus. Basically, the only exposure it has to the mother's world is through the placenta (afterbirth). This exposure essentially involves substances that are found within her bloodstream like oxygen and nutrients (and drugs, if used and absorbed). If the drug is not found in the mother's bloodstream during the first trimester when the baby is still forming its various body parts, then a drug-induced birth defect is very unlikely to occur. Therefore, **drug absorption is important along with the timing in the pregnancy**.

And The Baby Will Arrive When?

Before we proceed further into the topic of birth defects, we should discuss pregnancy dating. In most instances, the **due date** of a pregnancy (when the baby is due to be born), is based upon a woman's last menstrual period. This dating method is usually the case if the woman had regular menstrual cycles and she remembers or she wrote down **the first day of her last period**.

Ultrasound procedures have become a major part of obstetrics in the modern world and many pregnancies are now **dated** based on sonogram measurements (ultrasound and sonogram mean the same thing). It is important to note, however, that the dating of a pregnancy by sonogram uses the same principal as the first day of the last menstrual period.

Have I thoroughly confused you yet? Let me try to explain. A normal pregnancy lasts about 40 weeks from the first day of the last menstrual period to the due date (assuming the woman has menstrual cycles every 28 days without fail). However, most of you realize that you are not actually pregnant during menstruation. When a woman becomes pregnant, the conception (joining of the egg and sperm) occurs about 14 days after the first day of the woman's last menstrual period (again using the woman who has the perfect 28-day cycle). Therefore, pregnancy from the time of conception to the due date is actually 38 weeks. The reason 38 weeks is not used is because not all women know when conception occurred, but they usually remember the date of their last menstrual period. To explain this better, let's use an example.

Pregnancy Dating By Ultrasound

If a woman had a last menstrual period that started on August 1 (always use the first day of the last menstrual period), her due date would then be 40 weeks later or May 8 of the next year. If she were to become pregnant, conception would have occurred on approximately August 15 (again assuming a 28-day menstrual cycle). When seen by her obstetrical caregiver on September 19, she is told the pregnancy is seven weeks along which is seven weeks from the first day of her last menstrual period of August 1 (but she is only five weeks from conception). If an ultrasound is performed on September 19, based on the measurements of the baby, she is told the pregnancy is seven weeks along, not five weeks (see figure 2).

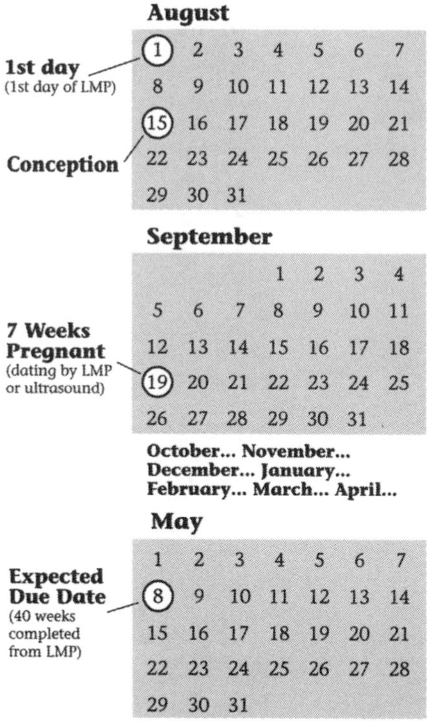

Figure 2:
This calendar displays a hypothetical case of a woman with a last menstrual period (LMP) that starts on August 1st. Conception would occur on August 15th (assuming ovulation occurs on the 14th day from the first day of the LMP). On September 19th, the patient is 7 weeks pregnant (but she is actually 5 weeks from conception). If an ultrasound is performed on September 19th, the patient is told she is 7 weeks along.

Later, when she is seen on November 21, she is told that the pregnancy is now sixteen weeks along (which is fourteen weeks from conception). Likewise, if a sonogram is performed on November 21, based on the measurements of the baby, she is told the pregnancy is sixteen weeks along, not fourteen weeks. As you can see, the ultrasound measurements automatically added in the two weeks from the first day of the last menstrual period to the time of conception. Therefore, dating a pregnancy by ultrasound and dating a pregnancy based on the last menstrual period have the same result.

Pregnancy Dating Through Fertility Specialists

Some of you may have become pregnant through the help of fertility specialists and will know the exact day of conception. However, your fertility doctor will still add in this two-week time period so that the due date will match the dating of women who used the first day of their last menstrual period or an ultrasound to date their pregnancies. Let's use another example to explain. If a woman has artificial insemination and four weeks later has a positive pregnancy test, she is told the pregnancy is six weeks along, not four weeks. Therefore, if a woman becomes pregnant through the help of a fertility specialist, the due date should be calculated as 38 weeks after the time of suspected conception.

From this point on in this book, if we discuss specific dates in a pregnancy, we are using the dates based on the first day of the last menstrual period or dates based on ultrasound measurements and not on the amount of time that has passed from the date of conception. The reason for this discussion is because your healthcare provider will talk with you during a pregnancy using dates based on the due date (which was calculated from the first day of the last menstrual period or an ultrasound) and, more than likely, will NOT be speaking about the number of weeks from the time of conception.

Another point women should know is that the due date is often called the expected delivery date or the expected date of delivery (EDD). It may also be called the expected date of confinement (EDC). (Don't you just love the word **confinement**? As you will probably notice during your pregnancy, many of the obstetrical terms used today were created by men.)

Creative Wording To Divide Nine Months By Three

A woman's pregnancy is often broken down into **trimesters** (three, 3-month time periods). The first trimester is from the first day of the last menstrual period up to weeks 12 to 13. The second trimester is roughly from weeks 12 to 13 up to weeks 24 to 26, and the third trimester is from weeks 24 to 26 to your due date (Dare I use the word confinement again?). Furthermore, it is also important to realize that your due date is not necessarily the **exact day** that you will deliver. The due date is used by a healthcare provider to help guide the management plan for a pregnancy. Comparing how far along a woman is at a specific prenatal visit to the size of the uterus can help determine whether or not the baby is growing properly. In addition, specific tests may be ordered at certain times during a pregnancy based on gestational age (how far along a woman is in pregnancy). He or she will also use the due date to prevent a woman from going too long before delivery. Yes, it is possible to go beyond the due date but usually a pregnancy will not be allowed to go much further than two to three weeks.

Ultrasound Dating—Not A Romance Between Technicians

Ultrasound can be a very good tool in dating a pregnancy if it is performed early in gestation (pregnancy). However, the farther along a pregnancy is, the less accurate ultrasound becomes in dating. For example, let's say that a pregnant woman has an ultrasound examination performed, and the results show that the pregnancy is 16 weeks along at that time. By using this information, she is given a due date of May 15. Her healthcare provider decides to have another sonogram performed 20 weeks later. Using the dates from the first ultrasound as the base, the pregnancy is now expected to be 36 weeks along (16 weeks plus 20 weeks). This next sonogram, however, shows that the baby measures to a 38-week size, suggesting a due date two weeks earlier or May 1. **It is very important to note** that she is still 36 weeks into the pregnancy and the **due date has not changed** to May 1 based on this second ultrasound. Her due date is still May 15 and the fact that the baby measures to a 38-week size only suggests that it may be larger than the average baby. (By the way, in the United States the average birthweight is about seven pounds, but who can determine what's average for you?)

Ultrasound dating has a plus or minus error factor in relationship to dating a pregnancy. This error factor varies based on when the ultrasound is performed during the pregnancy. If an ultrasound examination is obtained prior to 12 weeks' gestation, the plus or minus error is **only three days**. Therefore, a first trimester scan is very accurate in dating a pregnancy. However, if an ultrasound examination is rendered after 34 weeks gestation, the plus or minus error can be **up to three**

weeks. Therefore, late third trimester scans are not very accurate for pregnancy dating.

As you can see in the example above, when the pregnant woman had the second ultrasound at 36 weeks, she was at the time in her pregnancy when the largest margin of error could occur. Thus the earlier scan at 16 weeks was much more accurate in dating the pregnancy. This certainly is not to say that the second ultrasound has no value. Using information from the second ultrasound compared to the first can help guide management issues such as whether or not additional testing is needed or when delivery should occur.

Although an ultrasound examination is one of the tools that can be used during a pregnancy, not all pregnancies require one. In fact, specific guidelines exist suggesting when sonograms should be considered. If an ultrasound is performed, it oftentimes may be the only one required. Therefore, the example above was not to imply that every pregnancy will require two or more ultrasound examinations.

Drugs And The Issue Of Timing

Weeks One and Two

Now that you understand pregnancy dating, when discussing birth defects and their relationship to drugs, remember that the timing or the dates in a pregnancy are key points to consider. For the most part, birth defects will not occur if a drug or medicine is taken in the first two weeks of the pregnancy because the woman is NOT pregnant yet. In addition, no one has been able to prove that a medication can cause a problem in the egg or sperm that is then carried into the pregnancy.

Laboratory tests have been performed where the egg and/or sperm were altered or exposed to strong drugs. When this occurred, the egg or the sperm were no longer capable of joining together to form a conception. Furthermore, many men and women have been studied who have taken strong medications such as cancer treatments or have experimented with powerful illicit drugs such as cocaine, heroin, and marijuana, but stopped prior to becoming pregnant. When these women (or couples) became pregnant (and were no longer using the drugs) there was no higher rate of birth defects when compared to couples who had never used any of the drugs.

Week Three

Week three of the pregnancy is the first week after conception. In most cases, the egg and sperm join together in the fallopian tube (the passageway from the ovary to the inside of the uterus). Following conception, the embryo travels into the uterus and attaches itself onto the wall (a process called **implantation**) so it can obtain nourishment and oxygen for its development (see figure 3). Conception through implantation takes about five to seven days to complete. At this point the embryo only consists of about 32 to 64 cells, and the body parts and organs (such as the heart, brain, arms, legs, etc.) have not yet started to form. For most of this week, the embryo is not exposed to the mother's bloodstream and therefore is not actually exposed to drugs in any significant amount.

Week Four

The fourth week of the pregnancy is the second week after conception. During this week, some of the cells of the tiny embryo develop into what will become the placenta (afterbirth). These placental cells help the pregnancy attach more firmly to the wall of the uterus. The remaining cells start to develop into what will eventually become the baby (or the fetus). These baby cells basically evolve into three main tissue types. One form of tissue (the ectoderm) makes up the skin, brain, spinal cord, and nerves. The second tissue type (the mesoderm) makes up the muscles and connective tissue of the body, and the third tissue type (called endoderm) makes up the majority of the internal organs, such as the liver, kidneys, lungs, and intestines.

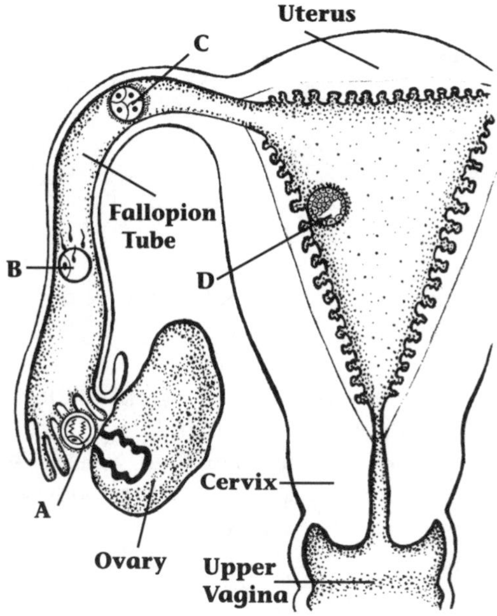

Figure 3: *This illustration shows a woman's female anatomy depicting ovulation, conception, and implantation.*

A. *The egg is ovulated (released) from the ovary.*
B. *Fertilization or conception occurs (when the sperm joins the egg).*
C. *The new conception begins to divide and is called an embryo.*
D. *The dividing embryo attaches to the inside wall of the uterus, a process called implantation.*

If a drug or medication were to significantly alter the embryo in weeks three and four, the entire pregnancy would usually be lost. This is called an **all or nothing effect** meaning the pregnancy would most likely either continue unharmed or would miscarry.

Weeks Five through Twelve

The most dangerous time period for producing birth defects usually occurs after week four up to weeks 12 to 13 in the pregnancy (which is more than two weeks from the time of conception). It is during this 8- to 9-week time span that the major body parts and organs of the baby form. From the following examples you will see why the first few weeks of this time frame are the most significant.

- The central nervous system (the brain and spinal cord) is the first organ system to develop at 4½ weeks and is basically finished by 10 weeks.
- The forming of the heart begins at 4½ weeks and is also basically finished by 10 weeks.
- The intestinal tract (the esophagus or tube from the mouth to the stomach, the stomach, the small and large intestines, and the rectum) starts to develop at about 6 to 7 weeks. The small and large intestines actually form outside the body of the baby, they rotate, and then move to the inside of the body by 11 to 12 weeks.
- The eyes and the ears start to form at around 5 to 6 weeks and are basically finished by 10 weeks.
- The arms and legs start to develop at about 6 weeks. They have an upper portion, a lower portion, and hands and feet by 9 weeks, and are usually complete with fingers and toes by 10 weeks.

- Shortly after the intestinal tract starts its formation at 6 weeks, the lungs bud off (grow off) of this and by 8 weeks have developed into the right and left lungs. However, these lungs are not capable of sustaining life until the pregnancy goes beyond 23 to 24 weeks' gestation.

The above list shows that the formation of the internal organs and the outside appearance of the baby occurs in the first trimester (primarily from weeks 5 through 12). The baby's remaining time in the uterus involves the finishing touches on some of the internal organs along with a maturing process of all the body parts so they function properly after birth.

Weeks Thirteen to Delivery

If drugs or medications are taken after the first trimester (after weeks 12 to 13) of the pregnancy, they are unlikely to cause major birth defects because the principal body parts and organs are already formed. Drugs will not deform a body part or organ once it is formed. They might, however, affect how body parts or organs function after birth.

Terrible Teratogens

As stated earlier, very few drugs or substances have been proven to cause birth defects. A few **teratogens** (drugs that cause birth defects), however, have been identified.

The first drug to be identified as a teratogen was thalidomide (thuh-LID-o-mide). Although this drug was used for many years by pregnant women, it was not until 1961 that thalidomide was found to be a problem. This medicine produced major deformities of the arms and legs in about one-third of the newborns exposed to the drug in the first trimester while in their mother's womb. It was prescribed for women (primarily in

Europe) as an antianxiety medicine (to help the mother relax) and to treat nausea. Unfortunately, it took several years and the birth of many deformed babies to identify thalidomide as the cause. However, the cause and effect relationship of thalidomide was one of the catalysts behind stronger drug regulations in the United States in 1962.

Another example of a drug that is a teratogen is an acne medication called isotretinoin (eye-so-TRET-tin-oyn) or Accutane (AK-you-tayne). This has been a highly effective drug for sufferers of severe cystic acne. However, if a pregnant woman uses this medicine during the first trimester, there is a very high incidence of birth defects of the brain, face, and heart. Therefore, if a woman has the potential of becoming pregnant (which is from puberty to menopause) and is prescribed this medication, before it is taken, **it is imperative** that she not be pregnant and that some form of birth control is implemented for the duration the drug is used. The medications, in the above two examples, require a prescription. **None of the over-the-counter drugs in this book have been proven to cause birth defects in humans.**

To Summarize

Remember, if a drug has the potential to cause a birth defect, it has to be taken after conception, it has to be absorbed into the bloodstream, it has to cross over to the baby from the blood flow in the uterus, and this usually has to happen during the first trimester when the baby is forming. A drug's role in potentially causing birth defects topped our list because it is often the number one concern of pregnant couples.

2. Drugs might cause one of the baby's organs to not function properly leading to damage somewhere else.

The second way a drug can affect a pregnancy is by acting upon an organ in the body of the baby causing it to not function normally. This, in turn, might lead to damage elsewhere. The best way to explain this is by using an example.

The Case Of The Overactive Thyroid

Some people have **overactive thyroid** glands which produce **too much** thyroid hormone. One of the ways to treat this condition is with a medication that slows down the gland's activity. This medication, if taken during pregnancy, can cross the placenta and possibly slow down the baby's thyroid gland as well. Although this sounds bad, the baby does not strongly require the function of the thyroid gland while it is in the mother's womb. The thyroid gland produces thyroid hormone, and this hormone helps in regulating our metabolism and plays a role in maintaining our body heat. The baby, however, is in a warm bath while in the uterus and this warmth is supplied by the mother's body heat.

The main active thyroid hormone in our body is abbreviated T3. In the forming baby, the thyroid gland produces something called Reverse-T3, an inactive hormone. The baby quickly changes to making normal T3 immediately after delivery. Therefore, once the baby is delivered, it needs a normally functioning thyroid gland because now it must maintain its own heat and essentially maintain its own metabolism.

If a pregnant woman was taking a thyroid medication (like the one described above) to treat an overactive thyroid gland, the baby could have a low thyroid hormone level after the delivery. If this drug usage was ignored (as far as her pregnancy was concerned), and if the baby was to have a low level of thyroid hormone for a long period of time after birth, this problem could lead to brain damage.

Why Would A Mother Do Such A Thing?

This above example was chosen because it explains how a drug which doesn't necessarily affect a baby while still in the uterus could result in damage after birth. This example would be unlikely to occur in the United States because all babies are tested for thyroid function after delivery. A low thyroid level in a newborn is a preventable cause of brain damage. You might wonder why a pregnant woman would take a medication that could harm her baby. The reason is that a woman who has an overactive thyroid gland can develop many other significant problems during a pregnancy that could result in an injured baby **if she were not treated**. Therefore, if thyroid function is too high and treatment is suggested, the risks of not treating the mother are probably higher than the risks of the drug itself.

On The Other Hand

Although thyroid problems are prevalent in women, the most common disorder is a **low level** of thyroid hormone. Therefore, many women take thyroid hormone replacements **to increase** their levels. You can be reasonably assured that if you are one of these women, the thyroid replacement medication is unlikely to cross the placenta and will have no effect on the baby. The example above involved an overactive thyroid gland producing too much hormone which is actually a rare disorder in pregnancy.

3. Drugs might lead to problems that show up later in life.

This is the most difficult area to study when considering the use of medicines during pregnancy. The best example of this was the use of diethylstilbestrol (dye-ETH-ul-still-BES-ter-all) which is commonly known as DES. This drug was given to an estimated six million pregnant women between 1940 and 1970. Its intended use was to hopefully prevent miscarriage, preterm delivery, and various other problems seen in pregnancy. However, it became apparent in the late 1960s and early 1970s that women exposed to this drug while in their mother's womb (these women are called DES daughters) had a higher risk for problems with their own vagina, cervix, and uterus. Some of these problems were an increased risk of miscarriage, infertility, and even an increased risk for a rare type of vaginal and/or cervical cancer. In 1971, the U.S. Food and Drug Administration (FDA) banned the use of DES in pregnancy. The majority of women who have suffered from DES-related problems were exposed to the drug in the first trimester.

This topic may still be confusing, so let's use another example. Let's say a woman becomes pregnant in 1950 and at six weeks into the pregnancy bleeding occurs. Her doctor prescribes DES in an attempt to prevent a possible miscarriage. The DES is taken, the pregnancy continues, and she does not miscarry. Eventually, she gives birth to a healthy daughter. The daughter, 20 to 25 years later (in 1970 to 1975), is found to have a problem with her cervix and uterus leading to pregnancy problems. She is the DES daughter. (A man exposed to DES in his mother's womb can have infertility problems; however, he is not usually referred to as a DES son—figures, doesn't it?)

The concept that a medication may cause a problem that shows up later in life is often a concern when talking about drug usage in pregnancy. However, the effect that was seen with DES does make sense. DES is a drug that is classified as a sex steroid hormone. In fact, our bodies actually produce their own sex steroid hormones. For men, the primary hormone is testosterone, and for women the hormones are estrogen and progesterone. DES primarily acts like a very strong estrogen, so it would make sense that the long-term effect was seen in the genital area of women and men.

4. Drugs might interfere with the function of the placenta (afterbirth).

The placenta is often called the afterbirth because in normal deliveries, the baby comes out first which is followed by the release of the placenta. The placenta is a round disc-like piece of tissue about eight to ten inches in diameter and about one inch thick and is attached to the umbilical cord. Some people have described the placenta as looking like a piece of raw hamburger meat. (This description is not meant to gross you out, but this is what has been happening in every delivery since the beginning of the human race.) The placenta interacts with the woman's uterus to supply the growing baby with nutrients and oxygen. The connection between the uterus and placenta is often referred to as the **uteroplacental** (utero for uterus and placental for placenta) blood flow. It is very important to understand that the blood of the baby and the blood of the mother do not mix. They are meant to be separate and should remain separate for the best possible outcome of the pregnancy.

Blood Flow Of The Baby

Starting with the baby, the blood that has already circulated through its body travels out through the umbilical cord to the placenta. In the placenta, it comes in close contact with the blood of the mother but **never mixes**. With this close contact, oxygen and nutrients found in the mother's blood pass across the walls of the blood vessels and enter the bloodstream of the fetus. The carbon dioxide and waste products (not urine or fecal material, but other used material) from the baby pass over to the mother for her to dispose of. Fresh rejuvenated blood then returns to the baby through the umbilical cord and is again circulated through its body.

Blood Flow Of The Mother In The Uterus

We just described the blood flow of the baby through the placenta. On the other side, the mother's blood enters the walls of the uterus by way of arteries (arteries are blood vessels with thick walls that carry oxygen-rich blood from the mother's heart to the various parts of her body). The blood in these arteries then flows into smaller and smaller blood vessels and eventually enters chambers called **intervillous spaces**. The blood vessels of the baby have looped into these spaces for the purpose of coming into close contact with the mother's blood. The mother's blood in these intervillous spaces then flows out and enters the veins of the uterus which eventually lead to larger veins outside the uterus and eventually back to the mother's heart to be pumped back through her lungs to get a new supply of oxygen. If you followed this description, you can see that the blood of the baby and the blood of the mother **never really mix** but only come in very close contact by passing each other (see figure 4).

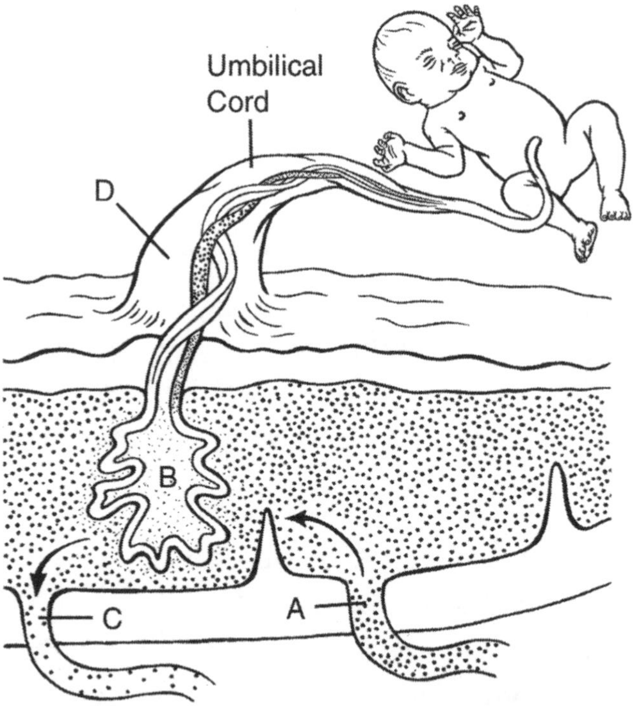

Cross-Section of Placenta

Figure 4: *This illustration depicts the blood flow in the placenta. The mother's blood and baby's blood should never mix.*

A. *Mother's blood flows into the placenta bringing oxygen and nutrients.*

B. *Baby's blood vessel is bathed by the mother's blood. The baby's blood accumulates the necessary oxygen and nutrients.*

C. *Mother's blood flows out of the placenta.*

D. *Blood vessels of the baby enter and exit the placenta from the umbilical cord.*

Back To Drugs That May Interfere With The Placenta

A good example of a drug that could interfere with the function of the placenta is not really a medication that would be prescribed. Cocaine is an illegal drug that is frequently abused by people. When this drug is taken, it causes a person's blood pressure to increase shortly after it enters the body. The cocaine causes an increase in blood pressure by constricting or narrowing the passageway of the arteries.

Picture a garden hose flowing with running water. If you step on this hose, you will notice that the hose from the faucet to your foot will become tighter because of an increase in pressure, and the amount of water flowing out the end will slow down. In this example, the hose was the artery and your foot was the action of the cocaine. Because cocaine could constrict the blood vessels (or arteries) going to the uterus, in theory this will decrease the blood flow carrying nutrients and oxygen to the baby in the same way your standing on the hose slowed down the flow of water coming out the end. For some babies the effect of cocaine is only temporary, so not all babies exposed to cocaine in the uterus are damaged. However, many are at risk and unfortunately can be injured.

The Blood Flows Grows

I want to discuss the mother's blood flow a little further. You may ask why? The answer is—this stuff fascinates me, and hopefully it is interesting to you as well. First, let's start with the entire blood flow of the body.

The amount of blood pumped out of the heart to circulate through a woman's body when she is **not pregnant** is about four liters per minute. A liter is just slightly more than a quart, so you can see that the average (this wording may get me in trouble since my wife tells me that no women are "average") female's heart is pumping a little more than a gallon of blood per minute. When she becomes **pregnant**, the amount of blood pumped by the heart increases over time to about six to seven liters per minute which is about one and a half to almost two gallons of blood per minute. Switching to the uterus, when a woman is not pregnant, the uterus has a blood flow of about 30 to 50 milliliters per minute (or about one to two ounces of blood flow per minute). However, when a woman becomes pregnant, the blood flow increases to 500 to 600 milliliters per minute which is about 16 to 20 ounces (or over a pint) per minute, and about 10 percent of all the blood pumped from the heart goes to the uterus during pregnancy—amazing, isn't it?

5. Drugs might interfere with labor.

Some drugs might affect the process of labor. In fact, many of you may know of a woman who experienced premature labor and was treated with medicines in a hospital in an attempt to stop the uterine contractions so the baby would not be born too early. These prescription medications have been studied for years in pregnant women and are believed to be very safe **under the supervision of a doctor**. They are given to women who are in premature labor and usually to women who are more than twenty weeks into their pregnancy. Therefore, they are used long after the baby is formed. Believe it or not, there actually are some OTC drugs that could affect the labor process, but this will be discussed later.

6. Drugs might interfere with how the baby adapts to just being born.

The newborn goes through many changes right after birth. To review briefly, the baby does not really need to maintain its own body temperature while in the uterus since the mother is already doing that. The fluid in which the baby floats (called amniotic fluid) is like a warm bath that maintains its heat from the mother's body temperature. In addition, while in the uterus, a baby does not have to breathe in order to get oxygen and does not have to eat for nutrition. The baby is receiving its oxygen and nutrition from the mother by way of the placenta and umbilical cord. However, when the delivery occurs, the newborn has to start breathing almost immediately in order to have enough oxygen, and now this little naked wet bundle of joy has to start maintaining its own body temperature. As you can see, a lot of things have to happen in the baby right after it is born.

Some drugs can affect how the baby functions right after birth. If a strong pain medication is given to the mother shortly before the delivery, that drug could sedate the baby or make it so sleepy that it might not breathe normally or deeply enough immediately following its delivery.

I'm not implying that all pain medications given during labor are bad, because giving birth is a very painful process for some women. Furthermore, the pain medications used in labor are chosen because they **wear off** fairly quickly so their effect on a newborn is usually very small unless given to the mother right before delivery. If you have further questions or concerns about this topic, please discuss them with your obstetrical caregiver. Usually pain management in labor is discussed at some time during the prenatal care process.

3. What Should I Know About Basic Genetics?

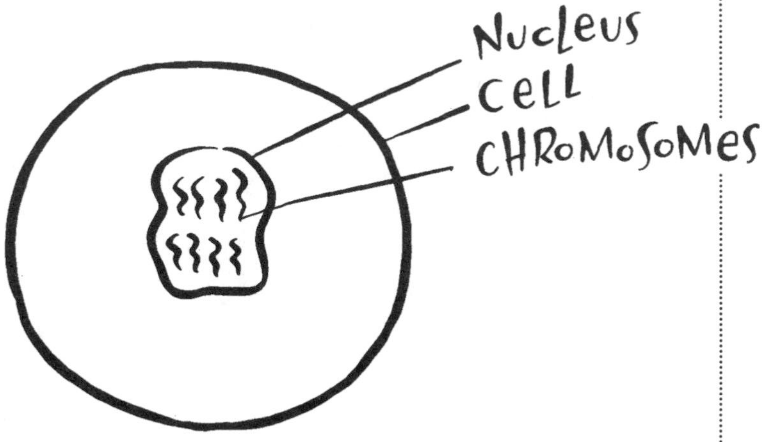

This subject is important because **most birth defects are caused by abnormal genetics and not by drugs**. Using a simple approach, genetic birth abnormalities can be divided into four basic categories. In explaining these four areas, we need to start with the word **chromosome**. Chromosomes are long strands of DNA that are found in the nucleus (center) of our cells. We use the abbreviation DNA because the actual words, deoxyribonucleic (dee-OX-ee-rye-bo-nu-CLAY-ik) acid, are quite a mouthful (not to mention conversation stoppers). The topic of DNA has become very popular in recent years because of its use in our judicial system to help identify or rule out suspects involved in legal proceedings.

Higher Math: 23 Pairs = 46 (Maybe)

For human beings, the normal number of chromosomes is 46. This means there should be 46 complete strands in the nucleus of nearly every cell in the body. These chromosomes are numbered 1 through 22 and are in pairs. There is also one pair of sex chromosomes. Thus (if you are following me), there are

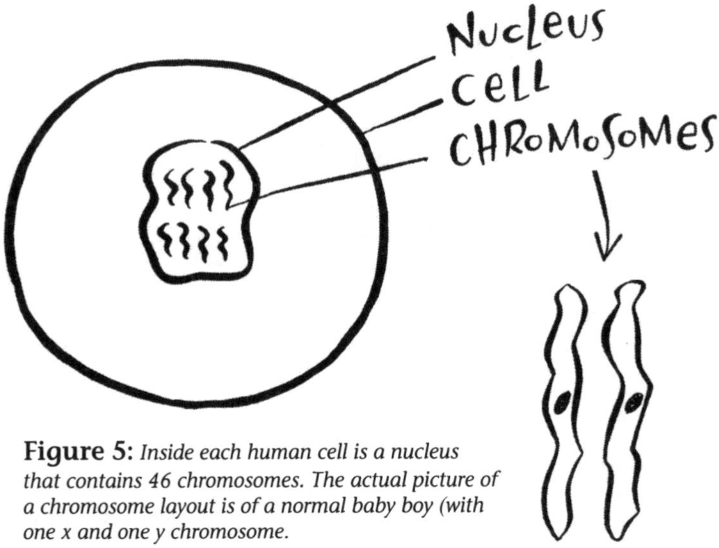

Figure 5: *Inside each human cell is a nucleus that contains 46 chromosomes. The actual picture of a chromosome layout is of a normal baby boy (with one x and one y chromosome.*

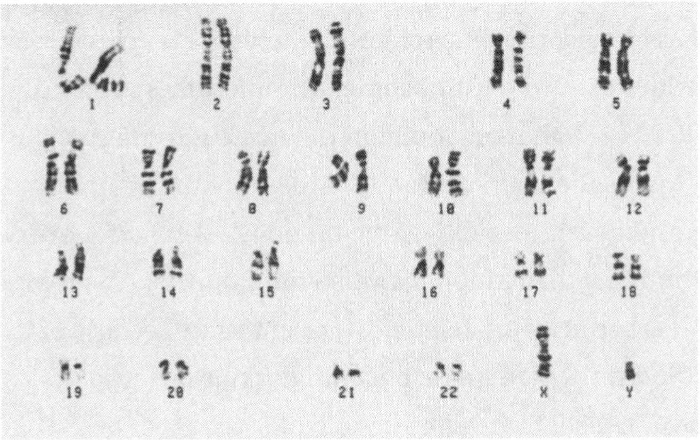

two number 1 chromosomes, two number 2 chromosomes, two number 3 chromosomes, and so forth, up to two number 22 chromosomes with one additional pair of sex chromosomes. These 22 pairs of chromosomes and the one pair of sex chromosomes add up to a total of 23 pairs or 46 individual chromosomes (see figure 5). Essentially all the cells in our body have 46 chromosomes except the egg and the sperm. The cells that eventually become the egg and the sperm start out with 46 chromosomes, but they go through a dividing process and end up with a single set of 23, which should be numbers 1 through 22 plus one sex chromosome.

Girls And Boys

The egg and the sperm both have one set of chromosomes numbered 1 through 22 and one sex chromosome. The sex chromosomes are labeled X and Y. If two X chromosomes are together, then you are genetically a female. If you have an X and a Y set, then you are genetically a male. Thus, each egg from a woman (if normal), has one set of chromosomes (1 through 22) with an X chromosome to total 23. The sperm from a normal male (perhaps **normal male** is an oxymoron, but bear with me) also has one set of chromosomes (1 through 22), but HALF of the sperm will have an X chromosome and the other HALF will have a Y chromosome. Therefore, if an egg which carries only an X chromosome, joins with a sperm that also contains an X chromosome, you will have a baby girl, because the child will have two X chromosomes. The chromosome count for this girl would be reported as 46 XX, which means she has a normal number of chromosomes in each cell (46) and, having two Xs, is a girl.

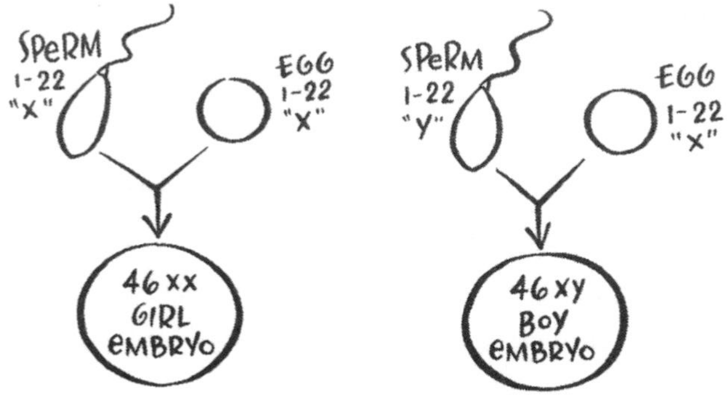

Likewise, if the egg joins with a sperm that contains a Y chromosome, you will have a baby boy. His chromosome count would be reported as 46 XY, meaning he has a normal number of chromosomes in each cell (46), and having one X and one Y, is a boy. You may have correctly figured out that every child gets one half of his or her genetic material from each parent.

Chromosome Abnormalities That Lead To Birth Defects

If a genetic birth defect occurs because of chromosomes, it could be caused by a person having too many chromosomes, missing a chromosome, or even missing a portion of a chromosome.

An example of a chromosome abnormality would be a person who has an extra number 21 chromosome. This person would have a total of 47 chromosomes instead of the normal 46. In addition, they would have three number 21 chromosomes instead of the normal two. The medical name for this abnormality is Trisomy 21 (tri which is the prefix for three and somy which is short for chromosome) but the common name for this condition is Down Syndrome. It is important to note that many other chromosome abnormalities can occur besides Trisomy 21.

The Needle Procedure

When you are pregnant, if you wisely choose to have prenatal care, some genetic discussion should occur with your healthcare provider. Depending on your age, family history, and whether you choose to have genetic screening (which will be discussed below) you may be offered the possibility of having a genetic **amniocentesis** (pronounced AM-nee-o-sen-TEE-sis). This procedure involves the placement of a very thin needle into the amniotic fluid that surrounds the fetus.

As you ponder this, you probably have surmised that the needle has to be inserted through the skin of the abdomen and through the wall of the uterus. As bad as this may sound, most women who have undergone the procedure report that the discomfort was minimal. In addition, the procedure uses ultrasound to help guide the needle into the fluid to avoid contact with the baby. The collected amniotic fluid contains cells that have fallen off the baby but are still alive. These cells can be studied and evaluated in a laboratory. After several days of preparation, the main test performed on these cells is to count the number of chromosomes and to make sure that no pieces are missing.

The purpose of discussing this procedure is that one of the major reasons for having a genetic amniocentesis is to identify chromosome abnormalities, and DRUGS DO NOT CAUSE chromosome defects. Another falsehood that has spread through society is that the amniocentesis needle is inserted through the navel (or bellybutton if you prefer). This is not true! The needle is never inserted through the navel because it is almost impossible to fully sterilize the depression. Usually, the needle is placed through the skin around the navel area.

Genes Not Jeans!

The next two genetic areas to discuss involve **genes**. Each of the 46 chromosomes can be broken down into smaller segments called genes. A gene is a small portion of DNA responsible for performing a specific function. Just as the chromosomes are paired up, as previously stated, each of the genes contained within those chromosomes are also paired up. It might be easier to explain this with an example.

At this time, geneticists don't exactly know which chromosome contains the gene for hair color. However, let's just assume that the gene for hair color happens to be located in chromosome number seven. If the person has a normal number of chromosomes (46), they would have two number seven chromosomes. Therefore, they would also have two genes for hair color. One gene would be on one of the number seven chromosomes and the other gene would be on the opposite number seven chromosome. Thus, as the number seven chromosomes are paired, the genes within each chromosome are also paired and the person would have two genes for hair color.

Because a gene in a chromosome is matched to a gene in the opposite chromosome, the words **dominant** and **recessive** come into play. The best way to explain this is with another example. If a woman with white skin has a baby with a man who also has white skin, the gene for skin color in the egg from the woman and the sperm from the man would indicate that the child should have white skin. When the child is born, the skin would be white.

However, if a woman with white skin has a baby with a man who has brown skin, the gene in the egg would suggest white, but the gene in the sperm would indicate brown. When the child is born, the skin color in most instances would be brown. This is because the gene for brown skin color is dominant and the gene for white skin color is recessive. Therefore, **for a recessive gene to express itself**, the gene on one chromosome and its partner on the opposite chromosome **both have to be recessive genes**. Whereas with dominant genes, only one needs to be present to be expressed in the child's makeup.

Four Possible Blood Types

Another good example for explaining the process of genes is blood types. There basically are four possible blood types: type A, type B, type O, and type AB. Blood types A and B are dominant, and blood type O is recessive. If an egg from a woman carries the gene for blood type A and the sperm from a man carries the gene for blood type O, when the egg and sperm unite, the child will have blood type A, because A is dominant and O is recessive. If the egg and sperm both carry the gene for blood type O the child will be blood type O because they are both recessive. If an egg carries the gene for blood type A and the sperm carries the gene for blood type B, the child will have blood type AB because both are dominant.

Some couples actually know their own blood types and the blood types of their children. It is possible for a woman to have blood type A and her husband to have blood type B but they have a child with blood type O. How can this happen? Well, we must remember that half of our genetic makeup came from our mother, and half came from our father. If the woman received an A from one parent and an O from the other, her blood type would be A, because A is dominant. However, remember that the cells that make up her eggs start with 46 chromosomes and end up with 23 which is half of the genetics. Therefore, half of her eggs would carry the A gene and the other half would carry the O gene. Likewise, if the father received a B from one parent and an O from the other, his blood type would be B, because B is dominant. However, half of his sperm would contain the B gene and the other half would contain the O gene. In the example above, this couple could have a child with blood type O, if the woman's egg with the O gene were to unite with the man's sperm that contained the O gene. Thus the child would have received two genes for O and would have blood type O (see figure 6). (I probably confused the heck out of some of you, but isn't this stuff great?)

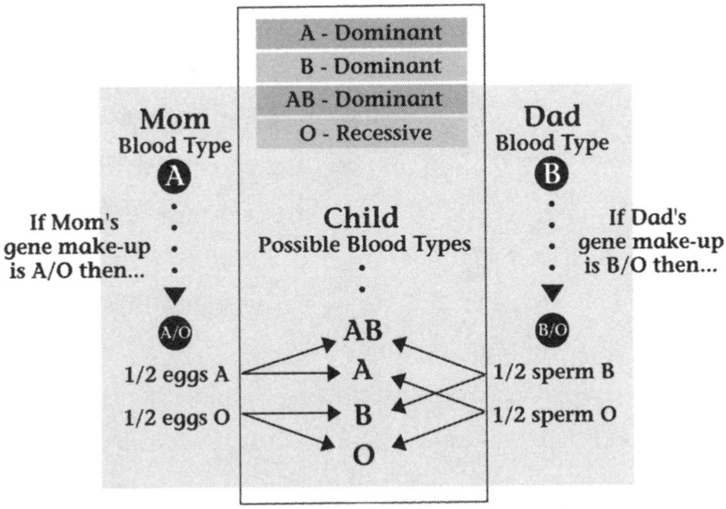

Figure 6: *Four blood types are possible: A, B, and AB are dominant and O is recessive. If a mom has blood type A (with a gene make-up of A/O and a dad has blood type B (with a gene make-up of B/O), they could have a baby with any of the four possible blood types. So, it is possible for a mother with blood type A and a father with blood type B to have a child with blood type O.*

In A Nutshell

Genes are either dominant or recessive. Furthermore, in most cases, for recessive genes to express their function, the pair of genes both need to be the same recessive gene, whereas a dominant gene only needs one to be expressed. As you may have guessed, some genes can be abnormal and they can lead to genetic abnormalities. If the abnormal gene is dominant, then only one is needed to cause the problem. This also means that only one parent may carry the abnormal dominant gene. If the abnormal gene is recessive, then the child has to receive this abnormal gene from both parents in order for the problem to occur.

Some examples of abnormal recessive gene disorders are Cystic Fibrosis, Tay-sach's disease, and Phenylketonuria (PKU). Some examples of abnormal dominant gene disorders are Adult Polycystic Kidney Disease, Huntington's Disease, and Marfan Syndrome.

After this discussion on dominant and recessive gene disorders, you need to know that DRUGS DO NOT CAUSE gene defects.

Many Factors May Be Involved!

The final genetic category to discuss is called multifactorial. As you can tell from the word, multiple factors play a role in this category. This part of genetics is very complex but for a birth defect to occur in this area, three major factors come into play: underlying genetic risk, timing in the pregnancy, and the environment. In addition, the majority of birth defects in this category involve the **structure** of an organ (for example, birth defects of the spine, the heart, or the upper lip, to name a few).

The Twin Example

Let's assume that identical twin sisters marry identical twin brothers. At this juncture, I need to explain the genetics of identical twins. Identical twins begin as one egg and one sperm that unite to form an embryo. However, very shortly after conception, the embryo splits in two, and you now have two embryos with the exact same genetic material.

Now, for the purposes of an example, let's say that the identical twin sisters both carry a genetic risk for cleft lip (a birth defect where the upper lip is not completely formed). As stated above, both of these women are married to identical twin brothers and they both decide to start their respective families. These twin sisters become pregnant at about the same time but they live in different parts of the country.

Unfortunately, one of the couples delivers a child with a cleft lip, whereas the other couple delivers a normal child. How can this be? To simplify a complex answer, the pregnant woman that delivered the child with the cleft lip was exposed to something in the environment that the other woman was not exposed to. In this hypothetical example, both sisters carried the same genetic risk for cleft lip, were both pregnant at the same time, but lived in different areas and were probably exposed to different substances in the environment.

The H-A-R-T Example

The example above is very simplified for a subject that is extremely complicated. It is highly possible that the underlying genetic risk in this multifactorial genetic category only occurs as a result of a combination of the genetics from the mother and the father, not just one parent.

Using another example, let's say that the underlying genetic risk for a birth defect of the heart requires a certain combination of genes that we will hypothetically label H, A, R, and T. It is possible that the mother could have all four of these genes in the egg, or the father could have all four in the sperm. It is also possible that the mother has the H and the A in the egg and the father has the R and the T in the sperm. When the egg and sperm unite, the fetus will now have all four genes. Therefore, many combinations exist that could result in a baby that has all four genes of H-A-R-T. Now, just because the fetus has all four of these genes does not mean that the child will have a heart defect. The fetus would have to be exposed to something in the environment at the time that the baby's heart was forming in order for the birth defect to occur.

Something's In The Air

It is also very important to define the **something** in the environment. The environmental factor could be a substance that is natural or manufactured. An environmental factor could also be a lack of something in the environment such as a vitamin or a mineral. These "somethings" which are present or absent might be found in the air or in our food. They also may be present for part of the time and absent for the rest, or maybe it takes a combination of several environmental factors to cause the problem.

Therefore, in most cases, the something in the environment is usually unknown and probably always will be unknown because the possibilities, as you can imagine, are endless. In addition, this environmental factor has to be present or absent at the time in the pregnancy when the particular organ or structure of the baby is forming and there needs to be an underlying genetic risk.

A Matter Of Timing

Using the example of the identical twins married to identical twins, let's say that both couples live in the same house and they have exactly the same diet. However, one wife becomes pregnant and then five months later the other becomes pregnant. Unfortunately, the first couple delivers a child with a cleft lip whereas the second delivers a normal child. More than likely, there was *something* in the environment that was either present or absent when the upper lip was forming in the child of the first couple that caused the cleft lip to form that was not present or absent when the upper lip was forming in the second child.

As you can see, both couples had the same underlying genetic risk and both lived in the same area, breathed the same air, and had the same diet. However, the timing of their pregnancies was different.

Back To The Multiple Factors

What is certain is that an underlying genetic risk must be present, and it must be combined with an exposure to something that is present or missing from the environment at the right time in the pregnancy when the particular organ or structure of the baby is forming in order for a birth defect to occur in the multifactorial category. Let's demonstrate this concept with a real-life example.

Spina bifida is a birth defect where the spine is not completely formed. The risk for this birth defect is about 5 per 1000 for an Irish person living in Ireland. For Irish immigrants coming to the United States, the risk drops to about 2 to 3 per 1000. The risk of spina bifida for a person living in the United States is about 1 per 1000 on the West Coast as compared to about 2 per 1000 on the East Coast. If a person from the United States which has a baseline risk of 1 to 2 per 1000 moves to Ireland, the risk may increase to 2 to 3 per 1000. As you can see, the highest risk is someone with Irish genetics living in Ireland, but the risk for this birth defect is not zero anywhere in the world.

The AFP Test

It is important to understand that all these genetic risks, for most couples, are relatively small and should be kept in perspective. Remember, using the example from the preceding paragraph, 995 Irish couples out of 1000 (or 99.5 percent) will NOT have a child with spina bifida. In addition, currently there is a screening test called Alpha-fetoprotein (AFP). This is a blood test that can be obtained from the pregnant mother when she is between about 15 and 20 weeks into the pregnancy. This test can screen for certain birth defects including spina bifida and can also be combined with other blood tests to screen for certain chromosome abnormalities.

However, if a pregnant couple seeks prenatal care after 20 weeks of gestation, there is little use for this screening test. If you want to have this test performed during your pregnancy, it is important that prenatal care starts as soon as possible once you determine or think you might be pregnant. In addition, some birth defects (but definitely not all) can be identified by ultrasound during certain times in a pregnancy. Again, ultrasound is also a very useful tool.

Some Final Words On Genetics

The topic of genetics is extremely complicated and we have only touched upon the surface of the subject. Other genetic syndromes exist that have not been discussed, but they are beyond the scope of this book. If you have a family history of a genetic problem or you just have more questions, it is highly recommended that you speak with your healthcare provider to address these concerns.

Finally, how do drugs or medications fit into this chapter? As you may have guessed, very little. Drugs or medications will NOT cause chromosome birth defects, will NOT cause dominant gene defects, and will NOT cause recessive gene defects. Therefore, a genetic amniocentesis is NOT indicated if someone has a concern that a drug or medication might have produced a birth defect.

However, drugs could be an environmental factor. Furthermore, if a drug or medication were to cause a birth defect, it would basically produce an abnormality in an organ or the structure of the baby. Therefore, the best screening tool for this problem would be a detailed ultrasound at the appropriate time in the pregnancy.

4. How Is Drug Safety Determined?

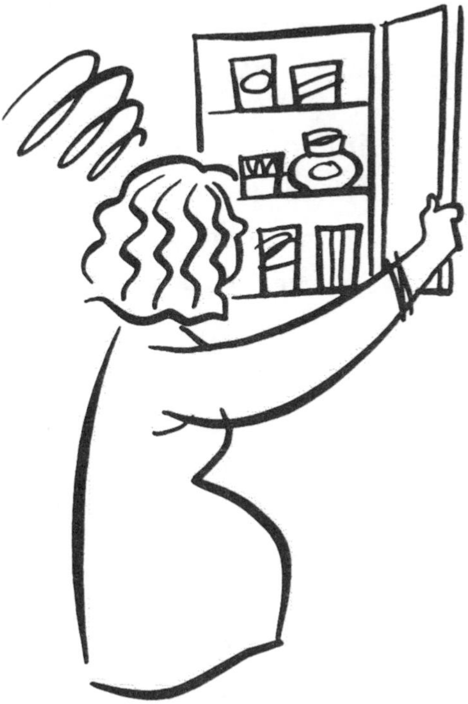

In all honesty, it is almost impossible to determine whether or not a drug is safe to use in pregnancy. The reason is because reliable studies cannot be performed during a woman's pregnancy to prove or disprove the safety of their use.

In order to conduct a reliable study that could answer this question, there must be a large number of pregnant women (let's say at least 10,000) who all live in the same area, are pregnant at the same time, breathe the same air, and have the same diet.

Then you would give one half of them a drug in the first trimester and the other half a placebo (a fake pill or sugar pill). After that you would need to follow them to delivery and observe the outcome. As you can imagine, this type of study never will be done and **never should be** done. At the present time, however, other less accurate ways are used to determine whether or not a drug is safe to take in pregnancy.

Epidemiological Studies

Simply stated, epidemiology is the branch of medicine that studies factors that may cause a disease or may influence the incidence of disease in large populations for the purpose of establishing programs to prevent or control the spread of the disease. One way in which drug safety in pregnancy has been evaluated is through epidemiological studies of human pregnancies. These cannot be well controlled which means that very few, if any, of the factors mentioned in the above paragraph are the same from one pregnant person to the next. However, these studies involve only humans.

Epidemiological studies are often conducted in one of two ways. The first is to evaluate drug usage in a random pregnant population (general pregnant population). The second method is to examine drug usage in a population of women who delivered children with birth anomalies or children with a specific birth defect.

Drug XXX—Where Can I Find Some?

Here's an example of a study involving the general pregnant population. Many women do not know they are pregnant in the early stages of a pregnancy. Let's say that a woman takes a drug called XXX and then a few weeks later she finds out she is pregnant. The pregnancy continues and she delivers a child. Researchers can identify this patient as well as other pregnant women who also took drugs during their pregnancies and attempt to put a study together. These researchers can then analyze those cases where the pregnant women took the drug in the first trimester, which is the time in pregnancy where birth defects primarily occur. Then they might compare these pregnancy outcomes to a group of pregnant women who never took the drug or they might compare the outcome to the baseline risk for birth defects.

As mentioned in Chapter 1, there is a baseline risk for birth defects in every pregnancy in the world. Remember, this risk is between two and four percent which means if you take 100 pregnant women who just delivered, two to four of the babies may have a birth defect. Fortunately, many of these are minor birth defects and do not affect the future of the child in any way. As I've said before, any time you deal with statistics, it is important to look at the values in the opposite direction, meaning that 96 to 98 of the delivered children will have no birth defects.

Many things are different between the pregnancies in an epidemiological study because the pregnant women live in different areas, are exposed to different substances in the environment, and have different diets. They also took the medication at different times in their pregnancies. However, these are the best studies available in considering the risk of a drug in pregnancy because they involve an analysis of the random pregnant population that has varying genetic risks.

The Second Way

The second type of epidemiological study evaluates a group of pregnancies that delivered children with birth defects. An example of this would be a study that evaluates first trimester drug usage in a group of women who delivered children with spina bifida (a birth defect of the spine). These studies may be helpful if they identify an unusual prevalence that is statistically significant for a specific drug. However, a group of pregnant women who deliver children with birth anomalies or a specific birth defect is a group of women who probably have an underlying genetic risk. These women **probably do not** represent the general pregnant population using the drug.

The Big Three

There are three substantial data bases that evaluated large numbers of pregnant women for drug use in early pregnancy. They are the Collaborative Perinatal Project (CPP), the Michigan Medicaid Surveillance Study (MMSS), and the Group Health Cooperative of Puget Sound (GHCPS) studies.

The Collaborative Perinatal Project[1] began in 1958 with the main objective of trying to identify factors during pregnancy or delivery that might play a role in cerebral palsy or other neurological problems seen in newborns. Information on drug usage during pregnancy was collected as part of the study. Later, this information was analyzed in regard to drug usage and the potential for birth defects. To date, the CPP is the most extensive and elaborate study of its kind. These data involve 50,282 mother-child pairs collected from January 1959 through December 1965 that were delivered at 12 centers in the United States. Every delivery (live-born or stillbirth) past 20 weeks of gestation was included. Each live-born child had several examinations after delivery and over 90 percent were followed for more than a year after birth. Extensive statistical evaluations were also performed.

The Michigan Medicaid Surveillance Study[2] was conducted by Franz Rosa, M.D., under the auspices of the Division of Drug Epidemiology and Surveillance at the U.S. Food and Drug Administration. Dr. Rosa was extensively involved in the research of drugs and their potential for causing birth defects. The MMSS is data collected from an online medical pharmaceutical analysis and surveillance system of Medicaid patients in Michigan. Information from two study periods was collected on various drugs used during pregnancies from January 1980 through December 1983 (104,339 patients) and from January 1985 through June 1992 (229,101 patients). A total of 333,440 pregnancies were recorded from both time periods. This study is different than the CPP because it involves data collected from computer-generated information. The MMSS could only analyze prescription drugs obtained as an out-patient and verification of use in all circumstances was not possible. This analysis could not collect data on drugs purchased out of pocket. Based on personal communication with Dr. Rosa, they determined through surveys that Medicaid patients were more likely to obtain drugs covered under the program than to purchase out-of-pocket medications. Unfortunately, Dr. Rosa passed away in 1997 before extensive statistical evaluations and verification could be performed. Therefore, only raw data exists regarding drug usage and outcome.

Information from the Group Health Cooperative of Puget Sound, Seattle, Washington is found in two publications[3]. These involve 13,346 women identified in the first trimester, many of whom used active ingredients contained in over-the-counter medications. The study period was from July 1977 through June 1982 and only included pregnancies that delivered live-born children. These data were also collected from computer-generated files and, therefore, verification of usage was not possible in all circumstances. Data on out-of-pocket drug purchases were not obtained. However, the GHCPS was a prepaid medical plan, and the vast majority of drugs were provided free or at reduced cost. This study included inpatient and outpatient prescriptions.

For those individuals interested in statistics, there are tables in the Appendix which compare the number of pregnancies with first trimester exposures identified in these three studies. The tables are divided into the various classes of drugs.

Case Reports

Another way in which drugs are analyzed is called case reports. These reports are about humans, but are limited to one pregnancy or at best only a few. In addition, these often involve cases where a birth defect was seen or a poor outcome occurred. Furthermore, these studies provide the numerator of the equation and not the denominator (for those of you who like math). In other words, is the risk of the drug (for causing that particular birth defect) 100 percent, or 50 percent, 10 percent, or zero? With a case report, no one knows.

Drug XXX Again!

To explain this further, let me return to the example where the woman took drug XXX and did not know she was pregnant. Let's say she continues the pregnancy and, unfortunately, the baby is born with a birth defect. This one case is then published in the medical literature. This would be a case report, but it does not give you the entire picture. What if an additional 99 pregnant women took the same drug in the first trimester but none of the babies delivered had that birth defect or any birth defect at all?

This would mean that the risk for drug XXX causing the particular birth defect seen in the case report was only one percent (1 out of the 100 pregnant women who took the drug in the first trimester). But, remember this one percent risk is lower than the baseline risk of birth defects of two to four percent in all pregnancies. Therefore, the birth defect seen in the case report more than likely has nothing to do with drug XXX. However, if nine of the additional 99 women delivered a child with the same type of birth defect, then drug XXX might play a role, because the risk would be 10 percent (or 10 out of the 100 women) which is greater than the baseline risk for birth defects. Thus case reports may be important for the purpose of future study, but they do not tell you what the present risk is for the drug or whether there even is a risk.

Animal Studies

The third way in which drugs are evaluated involves animal studies. These studies can be controlled because they are performed in a laboratory setting or in a confined environment.

Researchers take a group of animals (often mice or rats) and control the environment, the diet, and the timing of the drug exposure. One half of the animals are given the study drug and the other half are given no drug or a placebo. The animals later deliver and the offspring are examined for the presence of birth defects.

These studies are considered much better (from a scientific point of view) when compared to epidemiological studies or case reports, but how they compare to human pregnancies is poor in many respects. Many of these studies use large doses of the drug which would be way beyond any comparable dose that a pregnant woman would take. Furthermore, what may occur in a rat or a mouse may not occur in a human. A good example of this is the use of steroids during pregnancy.

The Case Of Steroids And The Pregnant Rat

The steroids I am talking about are used in the treatment of many medical diseases such as asthma, arthritis, and a disease called Lupus. (I am not talking about the steroids used to build muscle mass which have, in their own right, been associated with a multitude of problems.) The steroids that are given for the treatment of certain diseases have been used for years and studied in many pregnant women and no risk for birth defects has ever been identified. However, if these steroids are given to pregnant rats, there is a very high risk for cleft lip and palate (where the roof of the mouth and the upper lip do not form completely).

There are several reasons for the poor correlation between animal studies and humans. One of the most obvious is that humans are different than rats and mice (at least from a genetic standpoint). Furthermore, the placenta of an animal and the placenta of a human are different which may allow for a different passage of a drug from the mother to the baby when comparisons are made. (Remember, the placenta is also called the afterbirth and is the structure that attaches to the wall of the womb so that the baby can receive oxygen and nutrition from the mother while it lives and grows in the uterus.) The animal placenta may allow the drug to pass between the mother and the offspring, but the human placenta may not and vice versa. It is also possible that the placenta of the human may change the makeup of the drug before it passes over to the baby and the animal placenta may not and vice versa.

Knowing The Limits Of Drug Safety

As you can see, our ability to completely know how safe a drug is for use during pregnancy is limited. However, most drugs (prescription or non-prescription) that are available on the market have undergone some type of study using any or all of the three methods discussed above.

Some studies have been performed by the drug companies and others have been performed by outside researchers. When trying to find information on a drug's safety, you might read the Physicians' Desk Reference (PDR). Usually you will find a sentence under the pregnancy heading that reads something like "there are no adequate well-controlled studies in pregnant women, therefore this drug should only be used in pregnancy if the expected benefits outweigh the potential risks to the fetus." This statement is true because the study that is necessary to completely answer the question (as stated in the first paragraph of this chapter) cannot be performed in humans.

Rating Drug Safety By Categories

Drug safety categories or risk factor categories (A, B, C, D, or X) for pregnancy have been defined by the FDA. These risk factor categories are used to designate a level of potential risk to the fetus. The letter designations are usually assigned to a medication by the drug company, but not all drug companies do this. Your healthcare provider may have other textbooks that discuss drugs in pregnancy, and it is possible that these books also have given a risk factor category to a specific medication if one was not assigned by the drug company. The definition for each category is seen below, and for each, an example is also given.

A: Considered to be completely safe

As you can imagine, very few medications, if any, are labeled category A because it would require well-controlled studies in pregnant women who took the drug in the first trimester with no increase in birth defects occurring. Based upon the above discussion, this would be almost impossible to obtain. An example would be vitamin C in normal doses, and some of you may even argue that this is not a medication.

B: Felt to be safe

This usually means that several studies in animals and/or pregnant women (involving large numbers of patients) have shown no harm. An example would be penicillin.

C: Uncertain safety

This means there are no good studies in pregnant women, and there are either no studies in animals or the results of animal studies are questionable. An example of this is most drugs available on the market today.

D: Known to cause birth defects but may have a use in pregnancy

You may wonder how this can be, but here's an example. Some people have epilepsy or other medical problems that can cause seizures or convulsions. A medicine called phenytoin (fen-EE-toe-in) is often used to control the seizures so the person can hopefully maintain a normal lifestyle. If a woman who is at risk for having seizures is taking this medication and she becomes pregnant, there is a risk that her child could be born with minor or major birth defects. However, if she were to stop the drug to avoid this risk to her unborn child, and then had a seizure, the seizure might cause more significant problems than the risk of birth defects. Thus, this is a case where the risk of taking the drug may be less than the risk of not taking the drug.

X: Known to cause birth defects with no real use in pregnancy

Examples in this category are thalidomide (a drug that was used for treating anxiety and nausea in pregnancy but caused severe birth defects of the arms and legs) and isotretinoin or Accutane (a drug used for treating severe cystic acne but if taken while pregnant could cause severe birth defects of the brain, face, and heart).

Drug Safety Beyond Birth Defects

The majority of studies in the medical literature that have analyzed the safety of a drug in pregnancy have looked at its risk for causing birth defects. You should also realize that drugs can affect a pregnancy in ways other than birth defects. Therefore, drug safety needs to take into account other issues such as the amount of drug taken or the dosage, the duration for which the drug was or is to be taken (such as days, weeks, months, etc.), when in the pregnancy the drug was taken or is to be taken, whether the drug is absorbed into the bloodstream or not, how long the drug stays in your system once it is taken, and how the body breaks the drug down and rids it from the bloodstream.

Therefore, many issues need to be considered when talking about drug safety in pregnancy and many of these areas will be covered when you read about the individual medicines in later chapters.

A Little History Never Hurts

At this point, I would like to inject a little history about the U.S. Food and Drug Administration (FDA) and what this governmental agency has done in the area of over-the-counter drugs.

Drugs have been for sale to the general public for hundreds of years and you have all heard stories of traveling salesmen or faith healers selling the miracle drug. Unfortunately, the miracle drug could have been something simple like colored sugar water or might have been something addicting such as alcohol or opiates.

In 1927, the Food, Drug, and Insecticide (yes, you read it correctly) Administration was formed and initially tried to prevent people from being cheated by these traveling salesmen. However in 1938, an Act was passed and the focus of the FDA changed. Under the Act of 1938, drugs (both prescription and non-prescription) had to be proven safe before they could be sold to people for use. In 1962, amendments were made to the original Act of 1938. These amendments required that drugs had to be **effective as well as safe** before they could be sold to the public. In other words, the drugs had to do what they claimed to do and also had to be safe.

In the mid 1960s, the FDA began to review the thousands of drugs that had been approved since 1938 as safe for use by the general public (remember, the general public does not really include pregnant women). After the FDA had reviewed some 500 over-the-counter drug products, they found that only about one in four actually did what it claimed it would do. Thus the FDA decided that an extensive study of OTC products was indicated.

In the United States alone, there are an estimated 200,000 to 300,000 drug products available for sale to the general public. To review each one of these separately would take a few hundred years. Therefore, they began to evaluate the OTC drug products based on their active ingredients.

Several hundred active ingredients exist that, alone or in combination, may be used for many different health problems. In 1972, the FDA began its extensive review of OTC active ingredients based on classes of drugs, and over a period of time they developed monographs of their conclusions. To date, they still do not have final rulings on all of the OTC active drugs.

Over the past 25 years, several drugs have been removed from an OTC status because they usually were found to be ineffective. In the meantime, you probably have noticed that some drugs are now available for purchase over-the-counter that used to be accessible only by prescription. These drugs are often called switch drugs which means they have been switched from a prescription status to a non-prescription status (but usually in lower doses).

The FDA also reviews how over-the-counter medications should be labeled and what information should be given in the package concerning warnings and possible side effects. In conclusion, the FDA is still very active in trying to determine the safety and effectiveness of OTC drug products that are for sale to the general public.

II.

Part II.

Facts About Cold & Flu Viruses, Over-The-Counter Cold Remedies & Related Medications.

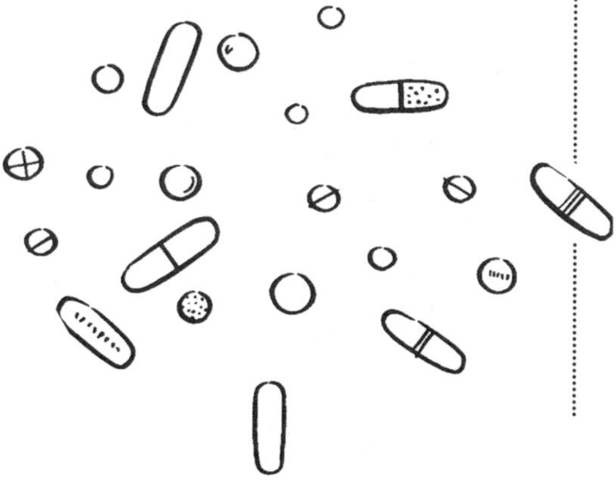

5. The Common Cold & The Flu

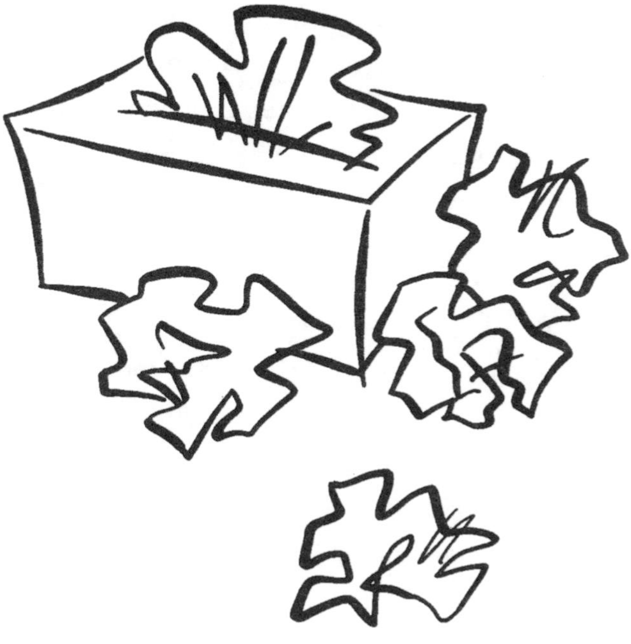

Unfortunately, developing an infection is something that almost everyone will eventually experience. Basically four categories of germs can cause an infection: bacteria, fungi (the plural of fungus), parasites, and viruses.

Bacteria

Bacteria are germs consisting of one cell. (Remember, a complete cell has all the parts necessary to multiply on its own.) Unlike most cells, bacteria may not have a distinct nucleus or center, but they do have genetic material (DNA). This genetic material is surrounded by stuff called cytoplasm which in turn is surrounded by a cell wall. Bacteria can multiply on their own, but to accomplish this, they use nutrients from the person they infect. Most bacteria can be killed with antibiotics, and some bacterial infections can often be prevented by using vaccines (injections which prevent diseases by stimulating antibodies against the germs). Some examples of bacterial infections are strep throat, staph infections, tuberculosis, diphtheria, tetanus, botulism, cholera, salmonella, and gonorrhea. A bacterium was also responsible for the devastating bubonic plague.

Fungus

A fungus is a germ which is also a complete cell that multiplies using a process called budding (a part of the cell branches out and develops into a new cell). These infections can be treated with antifungal medications which work like antibiotics by preventing the growth and reproduction of the fungus. Some examples of fungal infections are yeast infections, athletes foot, ringworm (which is not really a worm but a fungus), and others that can infect organs like your lungs.

Parasites

Parasites are germs that may have only one cell, but often consist of many cells. Parasites use the person they infect to help them survive and multiply. Some can be treated with antibiotics while others require different types of medications. Some examples of infections caused by parasites are malaria, toxoplasmosis (an infection transmitted by some cats), giardia lamblia (transmitted through infected water causing diarrhea), pinworms, tapeworms, and roundworms (these last three infect the intestinal tract), and African sleeping sickness.

Viruses

Viruses, on the other hand, are difficult to describe because they are not complete cells and do not have all the elements necessary to reproduce by themselves. They are similar to the nuclei of cells without the cytoplasm. In other words, they are made up of DNA or RNA, but they do not have a cytoplasm or cell wall surrounding them.

A virus has to invade a cell inside a person's body and then use some of that cell's materials in order to multiply. Since this book covers the over-the-counter drugs used for treating cold symptoms, it is important to know that **the common cold and the flu are both caused by viruses.**

The Common Cold

Rhinovirus and coronavirus are groups of widespread viruses which attack the respiratory system and are the ones most responsible for the common cold. Over 200 different viruses have been identified within the rhinovirus group alone. (The flu, on the other hand, is caused by different groups of viruses that each contain several members.)

In most cases, when a person becomes infected with a virus, a specific area of the body is attacked. For example, the hepatitis virus primarily attacks the liver, a stomach virus mainly attacks the intestinal tract, and the cold virus usually infects the nose, throat, sinuses, and bronchial tree.

Let's use one of the cold viruses as an example and assume that your body has just been infected. Because your body has never been exposed to this virus before, you have no immunity against it. Therefore, the virus quickly invades the nose, throat, sinuses, and bronchial tree. This invasion causes the tissue in those areas to become irritated, inflamed, and swollen. Furthermore, the virus will also kill some of the cells in these areas causing them to break apart releasing certain chemicals that further add to the irritation and swelling. This virus can also lead to pain in some of the affected areas. You now officially have the symptoms of the common cold: a stuffy, runny nose, full sinuses with pressure, sore throat, and chest congestion with a cough.

Our Immune System

As this process is occurring, your immune system (if it is working correctly) has now identified this cold virus as an enemy that needs to be killed. Therefore, it begins to develop antibodies to fight against the virus. The purpose of the immune system is to protect us from anything foreign such as viruses, bacteria, or even a foreign object like a small splinter.

At some time in your life, you may have picked up a small splinter after rubbing your hand across a piece of wood. Because the splinter was so small, you may not have noticed it was there. However, later that day or the next day you realize there is an area on one of your fingers that hurts. At closer inspection, you see a tiny splinter surrounded by a red inflamed tender area. Your immune system identified the splinter as being a foreign object that did not belong there. Therefore, it was trying to get rid of the splinter and, in the process, a reaction developed.

When the immune system identifies a cold virus as a germ that does not belong in the body, it starts creating **antibodies** for the purpose of killing the cold virus. Eventually, enough antibodies are produced, they kill all the viruses, and the cold symptoms disappear. In essence, you become cured! If you become re-exposed to the same virus at a later date, you usually will not get sick because the body's immune system already has antibodies that will kill it before it causes any problems.

However, if you are exposed to a different cold virus, you can become sick again because the body does not have a specific antibody to kill the new virus.

The Never-Ending Cold

When a person becomes ill with a cold, it usually lasts for about four to eight days and, barring complications, he or she will eventually get better. If a person has cold symptoms that last for three to four weeks, several explanations are possible. This person may have become infected with more than one virus in a sequential fashion, or he or she actually has allergies and not a cold. Another possibility is a secondary sinus infection that developed because of the cold.

It is also possible to be infected with two different viruses at the same time, which only makes the symptoms worse. It is important to note that many different viruses are passed between people during the "cold and flu season."

I'd Rather Catch A Baseball Than A Cold

The viruses that cause the common cold and the flu are spread from person to person through infected respiratory droplets. You can catch a cold by breathing the air after someone coughs or sneezes; however, the most common way people catch a cold is by direct contact. To better explain this, let's use an example.

Person A has a cold and sneezes into his or her hands. This person then enters a room by opening and closing a door. A few minutes later, person B enters the same room through the same door. To enter the room, both individuals had to touch the doorknob. The cold virus of person A was spread to his or her hand from the sneeze and then to the doorknob when entering the room. Person B then picked up the cold virus on his or her hand by touching the same doorknob. Person B could become infected by touching his or her eyes, nose or mouth while the virus is present on the hand. Maybe this is why our mothers always advised us to wash our hands before eating.

In a nutshell, cold and flu viruses are more often spread from hand to hand than through the air. Some of these viruses can live on hard surfaces for several hours. Despite what some people may say, you do not catch a cold from being exposed to cold temperature, or fatigue, or lack of sleep. You catch a cold by being exposed to a virus. From this discussion, you don't need to become paranoid every time you open a door, but good hand washing never hurts!

Pregnancy And Immunity

Because it is almost impossible to avoid exposure to cold and flu viruses, most pregnant women will catch a cold or flu at some time during their nine-month pregnancy. The possibility of a pregnant woman catching a cold or the flu is at least as high as anyone else's. However, are pregnant women more susceptible?

Studies have shown that the immune system may not be as effective when a woman is pregnant. The reason for this may be the baby. If you think about it, one-half of the baby is genetically different from the mother (because half the genetics is from the father). If the immune system were working properly, it should attack the baby because it is a foreign object. However, nature probably lowers the function of a woman's immune system to prevent this from occurring. Therefore, this weakened immunity may allow a pregnant woman to be more susceptible to catching a cold and it may take her longer to recover.

Protection Against Viruses

Although drugs that can kill viruses are available, most of these are very potent and are only used in certain circumstances. Therefore, the best approach for protection against viruses is to develop an immunity to them. There are two basic ways to become immune to a virus. One way is to become infected with the virus, as in the example above, where you suffer the illness as your body develops the antibody on its own. The second way is to be injected with **gamma globulin** or a **vaccine**.

Gamma globulin is an injection of actual antibodies that are directed against germs. However, over a period of time, these antibodies will disappear and you become susceptible again. A vaccine is a substance that can be given to a person causing their body to produce an antibody against a specific germ. Using vaccines is an approach that has been very successful, especially in dealing with viruses that produce a specific disease but have very few members in their viral group.

Smallpox Immunity

The best example of an effective vaccine was the one used against smallpox. This infection was responsible for killing millions of people worldwide. Smallpox was a virus that basically only had one member in its group. By vaccinating all people against smallpox worldwide, eventually everyone became immune. Therefore, because everyone had antibodies against smallpox, there was no one left to infect, and smallpox became extinct (so to speak).

Where's The Cold Vaccine?

Unfortunately, since the common cold can be caused by over 200 different viruses in the rhinovirus group alone, to make the common cold disappear, one would have to take so many vaccinations, the process would no doubt be worse than the cold itself. Furthermore, it is highly likely that we have not identified all the viruses that can lead to the common cold. Maybe this is why it is called **common**.

Antibiotics Cannot Kill Viruses

Another very important point to understand is that viruses cannot be killed by antibiotics. **Antibiotics kill bacteria**; however, most infections that people get, such as colds and flus, are caused by viruses. Therefore, you **do not need** an antibiotic every time you have a cold or the flu. Some people can become sick with a virus and develop a bacterial infection on top of it making them even more miserable. When this occurs, antibiotics can be helpful in fighting the bacterial portion of the infection.

To Prescribe Or Not To Prescribe — That Is The Question

The field of medicine is a confusing business at times. Some doctors feel that if they do not write an antibiotic prescription for patients who have a cold, these patients may not be satisfied with the care they received. So at times, doctors write a prescription for antibiotics that their patients may not need.

On the other hand, some patients always expect and want a prescription for antibiotics when they have a cold or the flu because it worked last time. You should understand that most viral infections last for about four to eight days. Usually, after about two to three days of feeling lousy, people decide to see their doctor for treatment. They receive an antibiotic and within two days of using the medication, they miraculously begin to feel better! In most cases, they would have started to feel better anyway without the antibiotic because the two to three days prior to seeing the doctor plus the two days after the visit equals about five days, which is when the viral infection would be going away on its own.

The Risk Of Antibiotic Overuse

What is the harm in using antibiotics too frequently? The main concern with taking antibiotics (especially when they are not indicated) is the possibility that some bacteria will become resistant over time. This means that the antibiotic becomes ineffective. With so many different antibiotics available today, this would not seem to be a serious problem. This statement is partly true and partly false. Well over a hundred different antibiotics exist on the market today. However, medications or drugs are organized into various drug classifications. Let me give you an example.

Penicillin is a drug classification which includes antibiotics such as penicillin G, penicillin VK, ampicillin and amoxicillin. When a bacterium becomes resistant to one of the penicillin drugs in the classification, it is usually resistant to most of the penicillins.

All antibiotics used today can be classified into about 20 categories. Some antibiotic categories have only one drug member (an example is an antibiotic called clindamycin). Other antibiotic categories, like penicillin, have several different members.

In the early 1900s, the most common cause of death was bacterial infections, with pneumonia and tuberculosis heading the list. The discovery of antibiotics greatly impacted the advancement of medicine. Unfortunately, with the extensive and sometimes needless antibiotic usage over the past 40 to 60 years, some bacteria have developed resistance. In fact, news about resistant strains of bacteria are becoming very common in the current medical literature. Some of these reports include antibiotic-resistant strains of tuberculosis, pneumococcus, haemophilis, salmonella, and enterococcus (these words are a mouthful but they are names of real bacteria that are developing resistances). This serious problem has developed because of the widespread and extensive use of antibiotics.

Talking about potential future effects of resistant bacteria is similar to talking about future effects of pollution. You may not see the total picture right here and now, but these issues could be devastating in the future.

It is imperative, therefore, that you DO NOT expect your doctor to give you antibiotics every time you catch a cold, and be sure to let him or her know that this is okay with you. This isn't to suggest, however, that you should not consult your doctor if you have an unusually bad cold or flu. Bacterial infections can sometimes be involved, and specific findings in your examination may lead to the conclusion that the use of an antibiotic could be beneficial. I realize that it may seem like I am preaching on a soapbox, however, the issue of antibiotic overuse is important for our future and the future of our children.

What Is The Flu?

Above, we discussed the findings of the common cold, but what exactly is the flu? The term flu has become a catch-all term for viral infections that involve the respiratory tract (nose, throat, bronchial tree, and lungs). Usually the common cold bothers the nose, sinuses, and throat, more than the bronchial tree, and fevers are usually low grade and mild.

However, the viruses that cause the flu usually affect the bronchial tree and lungs, and the fever is often higher. In addition, flu symptoms include headaches, muscle aches, and a general overall lousy, rotten, and run-down feeling. Most of us have had the flu at some time in our life, and hopefully I have described the symptoms to most people's satisfaction. In addition, as you may have already determined, there is an overlap between the common cold and the flu.

Some people also use the term flu for infections that can cause a stomachache, nausea, vomiting, and diarrhea. Indeed, there are viruses that can infect the intestinal tract, but most people call these a stomach virus or stomach flu.

Fevers

When a person has a fever, they usually do not feel well. However, a fever is produced by the body as a means to combat, slow down, or kill an infection. In other words, the fever is part of the body's defense mechanism. Therefore, not all fevers are bad and, in some respects, a fever may help fight the infection. What is important is how high the fever is and this should be discussed with your healthcare provider.

When talking about a fever in pregnancy, however, we also have a fetus in the uterus experiencing this temperature and the management is more complicated. Some experts feel that any fever in pregnancy might cause a problem for the unborn baby and thus recommend treatment. However, other experts suggest treatment for only high fevers. The subject of fevers in pregnancy is an area that you should discuss with your healthcare provider, especially if one develops. Aside from a cold or flu, a fever may be telling you that something is wrong and you should find out what it is.

In The Final Analysis

If you become ill with a cold or flu, and have been feeling rotten for two or three days, remember that you might only have to ride it out for a few more days before your body's defense system cures the problem.

If you have concerns or questions, you should always call your healthcare provider to seek his or her opinion about whether or not an office visit is warrented. When the so-called "cold and flu season" is here, you may become even more sick by exposing yourself to more germs in the doctor's office! Think about it.

6. Ingredients Found In Cold Remedies

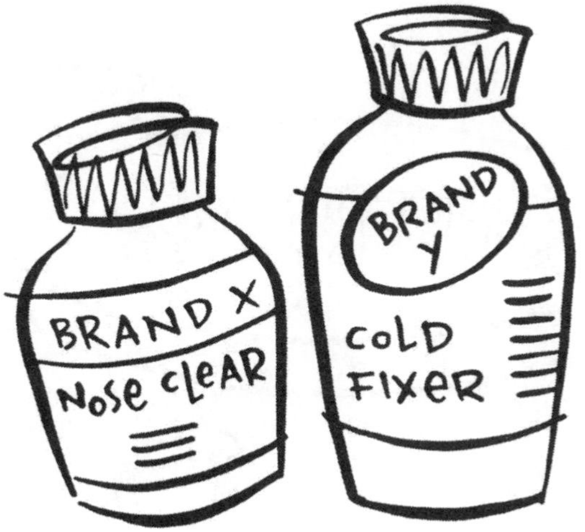

What are cold remedies? Well, this is a very good question. To begin with, these medications are not cures for the common cold or the flu, but instead they contain active ingredients that, at best, try to relieve the symptoms. There are many different ways you can be bothered by a cold (a runny nose, a stuffy nose, full sinuses with pressure, headache, fever, muscle or body aches, sore throat, chest congestion, and coughing). Therefore, OTC cold and flu medications contain drugs that can only try to minimize some of the above symptoms or at least make them less severe. You should also know that there is no single medication that can attack all of the symptoms. In fact, a single drug usually only attacks a single symptom.

At this point, remember that when I use the word drug, I am talking about one active ingredient. I am not talking about trade names or brand names. Over-the-counter medications often contain more than one active ingredient. Let me use a fictitious example.

"Superduper Cold Fixer" — The All-purpose Cold Remedy

Let's say there's an over-the-counter medication called "Superduper Cold Fixer." This pill can treat all your symptoms. It will alleviate your stuffy nose, sinus pressure, headache, sore throat, and cough all at the same time. "Superduper Cold Fixer" is only one pill, BUT it contains four active ingredients. These active ingredients are actually individual drugs. There is one that works on the nose and sinus area, another treats the headache, a third works on the cough, and the final drug handles the sore throat. Therefore, "Superduper Cold Fixer" consists of an active ingredient for each of your symptoms.

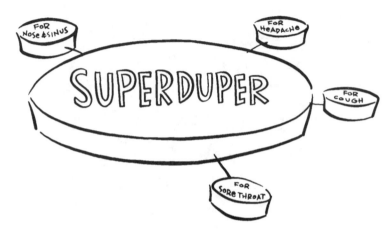

It may seem from the above discussion that I am not a fan of all-in-one cold remedies. On the contrary, to be able to take only one pill for all those symptoms is convenient, and on occasion, I have used them for my colds. However, all-in-one cold remedies are good only if a person has all the symptoms listed on the label.

If an individual has only one or two symptoms, he or she might be able to tailor which over-the-counter cold medication is purchased. This last statement becomes very important, especially if you are pregnant. The goal during pregnancy is to **use only what is needed**. Thus, the all-in-one cold remedies are not a good recommendation for most pregnant women.

OTC Cold Remedies Primarily Contain The Following Types Of Drugs

Decongestants try to un-stuff the nose and decrease sinus pressure (see Chapter 7).

Antihistamines are difficult to explain, but simply speaking, they work on allergy symptoms and may help alleviate a runny nose (see Chapter 8).

Expectorants are a misnomer, but they work by making the thick mucus or phlegm (Why isn't this word spelled flem like it sounds?) in the nose, sinuses, and bronchial tree a little thinner so the body can get rid of it easier (see Chapter 9).

Cough Suppressants try to help minimize coughing (see Chapter 10).

Others may include medicines for pain, medicines called drying agents, and caffeine (yes, caffeine).

As you can see, over-the-counter cold remedies may contain several different drugs. You also need to remember that when there are active ingredients, there are usually inactive ingredients. Inactive ingredients may include sugar, artificial sweeteners, alcohol, preservatives, lubricants, artificial colors, and different flavorings. The word inactive is also somewhat of a misnomer because all these substances have some function. They just do not work towards relieving the symptoms of a cold. When you buy a cold remedy (or any over-the-counter medication), you should always read the label that lists both the active ingredients and the inactive ingredients. Some of the inactive ingredients might surprise you.

For example, an over-the-counter cold medication may list aspirin and caffeine as inactive ingredients. The inactive ingredient section is the one that will list whether or not a medication contains sugar, artificial sweeteners, or alcohol. Knowing the active and inactive ingredients of a medicine can be very important for pregnant women and for anyone who may have medical problems such as diabetes, hypertension (high blood pressure), heart disease, allergies, or phenylketonuria (a metabolism disorder). You may wonder why these other ingredients are found in over-the-counter medications, but you will have to wait until Chapter 11.

7. Decongestants

Decongestants are a group of drugs used to unstuff your stuffy nose! Believe it or not, this class of drugs is probably **the strongest group** of over-the-counter medications you can buy for treating some of your cold symptoms. This is discussed in more detail in the section called The Crux of the Matter (pages 99-106). However, PLEASE—PLEASE—PLEASE read the next few pages before you turn to the individual drugs.

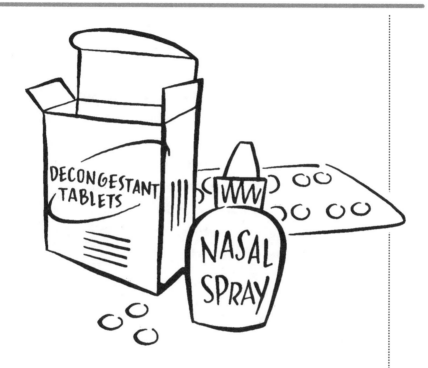

There are several ways of describing what these medications may do when taken. The FDA actually has regulations on the wording drug companies may or may not use on their labels! Here are some examples of approved wording: unclog your nose, help clear nasal passages, reduce swelling of membranes or shrink swollen membranes in your nose, help open sinus passages, relieve sinus congestion, relieve pressure in your sinus area, and restore freer breathing.

It is very important that you realize the above descriptive effects are only temporary. Furthermore, these drugs may help relieve some of the above symptoms for most people but may do nothing for others suffering from a stuffy nose or sinus pressure. You should also remember that these medicines only treat symptoms; they are not cures. Before you take any decongestant medication, be sure to read (and heed) the information found under the boldfaced sections below.

WARNINGS

Before using any OTC decongestant medication, persons with any of the following health problems should talk to their healthcare provider first.

- Heart disease
- High blood pressure
- Diabetes
- Overactive thyroid gland
- Narrow-angle glaucoma
- Kidney problems
- Liver problems

Reasons for these warnings are explained in detail in the section called The Crux of the Matter. If you have one or more of the above medical problems, using a decongestant could cause serious side effects. For some of you, it may still be possible to use a decongestant, but only after your healthcare provider says it is safe to do so.

A Disease Just For The Pregnant Woman

These warnings are especially important for pregnant women. A special type of high blood pressure called **toxemia** can develop during a pregnancy. Other names for this disease are **pre-eclampsia** or **pregnancy induced hypertension**. Most women of childbearing age have normal blood pressure and will continue to have normal blood pressure during pregnancy. However, a few women will develop hypertension while pregnant and this problem is called toxemia. This is one of the many things your healthcare provider checks for at nearly every prenatal visit. You should be aware that if you have high blood pressure very early in the pregnancy (in the first trimester), you probably had high blood pressure prior to becoming pregnant.

Too Much Protein

At most prenatal visits, your urine is tested to search for the presence of excess protein. If protein is detected at a certain level, this could be a warning sign that toxemia might be developing. If protein is found in the urine, this does not mean that toxemia has developed for certain. Its presence only suggests that further evaluation may be needed.

Too Much Sugar

In testing your urine, the presence of glucose (sugar) is also sought. Glucose in the urine may signal the possibility that diabetes is developing. You guessed it! Diabetes is another problem that can occur just because a woman is pregnant. This type of diabetes is usually called **gestational diabetes** because it only develops during pregnancy.

Gestational diabetes usually goes away after the baby is delivered. However, research has shown that nearly one-half of the women who have gestational diabetes will develop full-blown diabetes sometime within the next 20 years of their life. This future risk is probably related to a woman's weight, lifestyle, and diet.

You should know that many women spill sugar in their urine **just because** they are pregnant, but many of these women do not have gestational diabetes. If your urine is positive for sugar, your doctor will probably do a specific blood-screening test for diabetes. Therefore, if sugar is found, it only suggests that further testing may be necessary. However, if you have high blood sugar very early in the pregnancy (in the first trimester), you may have had diabetes prior to becoming pregnant.

Toxemia and gestational diabetes are conditions that usually develop or are seen in the second half of pregnancy (after 20 weeks). Therefore, since decongestants may be a problem if used by people with high blood pressure or diabetes, before using one of the active ingredients in this category, be sure that you do not have toxemia or gestational diabetes.

Drug Interactions

If you are already taking a drug, whether it is prescription or over-the-counter, that drug might react with or interact with the decongestant you are about to take and this could lead to problems. Furthermore, if you are not taking anything now but plan to use a new prescription with an over-the-counter decongestant, please read this section carefully. Remember that many over-the-counter cold remedies may have more than one active ingredient so be very careful if you plan to use more than one OTC drug at a time. Again, read the labels!

The categories below contain many of the drugs to watch out for.

• Drugs that are monoamine oxidase (MAO) inhibitors

MAO inhibitors are used for treating depression, other psychiatric and emotional disorders, and conditions like bulimia and panic attacks.

• Drugs that treat high blood pressure

If you are taking a high blood pressure medication, then you have a diagnosis of high blood pressure (even if your pressure is normal because you are taking the drug). Decongestants have the potential for counteracting the effect of the high blood pressure medication, which could result in the blood pressure becoming elevated again.

• Drugs that act similarly to decongestants

These could be medications used to raise your blood pressure if you have low blood pressure or using two decongestants at the same time. This issue is very important because if you take a decongestant pill and also use a nasal spray at the same time, you could end up over-medicating on decongestants. Therefore, if you plan to take pills for some of your cold symptoms along with a nasal spray to unclog your nose, be sure there is no overlap.

• Drugs that cause blood vessels to constrict (shrink)

Some prescription drugs are used specifically to constrict blood vessels (like some medications used for treating migraine headaches). Again, using a decongestant while taking those medications could lead to problems.

• Drugs that treat depression

Most of the categories listed above are prescription drugs. However, if you are taking any medicine (whether it is prescription or not), before using an over-the-counter drug, talk to your healthcare provider to be sure there is no conflict. (You may become tired of reading about this concept, but it is imperative that you read labels and/or check with your healthcare provider before taking medications concurrently—your life may depend on it!)

Two Sides Of Side Effects

Minor Side Effects

Some minor side effects that may be experienced while taking an over-the-counter decongestant (pills, nasal spray, nose drops, or nasal jellies) include:

- temporary discomfort in the nose such as burning, sneezing, stinging or an increase in discharge from the nose, primarily seen when using nasal sprays, nose drops, or nasal jellies

- nervousness or anxiety (heart rate may increase or a person may feel like their heart is pounding harder)
- insomnia (difficulty in falling asleep) if used too close to bedtime
- nausea or stomachaches after medications are swallowed (including liquids from nasal sprays and nose drops that may reach the back of the throat)
- headaches

Major Side Effects

The two major side effects that can occur when using over-the-counter decongestants are heart problems and high blood pressure. These serious side effects are usually seen in people who are taking more than the recommended dose printed on the label, are using it more frequently than what is recommended, or have just plain overdosed on the drug. Most people who use these medicines and follow the directions should not experience major problems.

Although rare, some individuals may respond differently to a medication at the recommended dose (or even lower than the recommended dose) based upon an unusual personal reaction. To identify these people before they use the drug is essentially impossible. In addition, prolonged use of decongestant medications could lead to a dependence, so the recommended period for usage is normally limited to a few days.

As If Your Life Depends On It!

If any of the following symptoms develop, you should stop taking the medication and contact your healthcare provider immediately:

- chest pain
- fast, pounding, or irregular heart beat
- wheezing or shortness of breath
- hallucinations (seeing or hearing things that other people do not see or hear)

If you start experiencing any of the following symptoms, I strongly recommend that you talk to your healthcare provider before taking the medication again:

- nervousness
- dizziness
- trouble sleeping
- nausea or upset stomach
- headache
- or any other feeling you think might be caused by the drug

The Bottom Line

The current list of available decongestant active ingredients found in over-the-counter cold remedies is as follows:

1. Oxymetazoline: nasal sprays, nose drops, and nasal jellies
2. Xylometazoline: nasal sprays, nose drops, and nasal jellies
3. Naphazoline: nasal sprays, nose drops, and nasal jellies
4. Propylhexedrine: nasal sprays, nose drops, and nasal jellies
5. Phenylephrine: pills and also nasal sprays, nose drops, and nasal jellies

6. Pseudoephedrine: pills only
7. Phenylpropanolamine: pills only
8. Levmetamfetamine: nasal sprays

If my wife were pregnant and she and I and our doctor decided to use a decongestant for several days during the pregnancy, I would choose No. 6 or 7 above (pseudoephedrine or phenylpropanolamine) based on how they work. Nos. 1 through 5 and 8 are basically **alpha drugs** while Nos. 6 and 7 are **both alpha and beta** in action (explained in The Crux of the Matter, pages 99-106).

The nasal spray products are only marketed with active ingredients that are primarily alpha in action. In an uncomplicated pregnancy, using these sparingly and sporadically at the recommended doses and frequency would probably be acceptable, but check with your healthcare provider to be sure.

The decongestants are a class of drugs where reading the directions and following them completely becomes extremely important, **especially if you are pregnant**! Since this book may be used as a reference guide, some information given about each individual drug may be repeated because all of the decongestants have similar actions.

Decongestants can be bought over-the-counter in the form of nasal sprays, nose drops, nasal jellies, or as pills (tablets or capsules). As you may remember from the first chapter, you will have to remove the over-the-counter cold remedy from the shelf and read the label or box to find one of the active ingredients listed above.

A complete list of active ingredients found in OTC cold remedy medications is located in the back of this book (Chapter 16) with references about their drug category and the pages where they can be found. Also remember that several drug names are very similar (with lots of letters), so be sure that you are looking for the same active ingredient on the package as the drug listed in this book. Furthermore, you should also read the inactive ingredient list (see Chapter 11).

Pregnancy And The Stuffy Nose

Nasal congestion unrelated to a cold or flu is common for some women during pregnancy. The reason for this may be that blood vessels are more dilated (open) when a woman is pregnant. Thus, if blood vessels are more dilated in your nose, you may have the feeling of a stuffy nose while pregnant, and this problem could last for weeks, and even months, at a time.

The Shrinking Straw

Nasal sprays, nose drops, and nasal jellies work by constricting blood vessels in the nose and possibly in the sinus areas. When reading about constricting blood vessels, picture a straw (that you drink through) and a piece of uncooked spaghetti. The straw has a larger diameter (is fatter) than the piece of uncooked spaghetti. Therefore, the straw would represent a swollen dilated blood vessel, and the piece of uncooked spaghetti would represent a constricted blood vessel. So when we talk about blood vessels constricting, think of the straw shrinking down to the size of the uncooked spaghetti.

When blood vessels in the nose and sinus area shrink, the swollen membranes also become smaller allowing air to flow through the nose easier and possibly lessening the pressure in the sinus area. Hence, the symptoms of a stuffy, clogged nose with sinus pressure often improve following the use of a decongestant.

Once Again, More Is Not Better

As stated in the beginning of this chapter, the amount of drugs taken and the frequency with which they are used as described on the product's label should be followed to the letter, especially if you are pregnant. (Sometimes detailed information is located in a package insert rather than on the outside of the package itself.) Nasal sprays, nose drops, and nasal jellies often produce rapid relief and breathing easier occurs fairly soon after usage; but this effect wears off over time. This wearing off may result in a person repeatedly using the drug in order to continue breathing easier. Unfortunately, in only a matter of days, the effect of the drug in many people wears off faster with each use. This may result in the person using the medication more frequently, leading to problems of overuse. This overuse can result in **rebound congestion** where the nasal stuffiness becomes greater than it was after the drug wears off, which then only makes the symptoms seem worse. This is the reason the package information warns you NOT to use nasal sprays, nose drops, or nasal jellies for longer than three days and to follow the recommended dosage and schedule exactly.

Don't Spread It Around

Because nasal sprays and nose drop applicators usually touch the nasal area they should **only be used by one person** to prevent the spread of infection. You're not being kind by sharing—one whiff from your nasal spray could cause days of misery for someone you tried to help.

Pills, Tablets, Or Capsules

Decongestants taken by mouth are usually absorbed into the bloodstream quickly, but there does not appear to be a risk for rebound congestion as seen with nasal sprays. Therefore, they can be used for a few days longer. Some researchers question the effectiveness of nasal sprays, nose drops, and nasal jellies in decreasing the pressure sensation in the sinus area. It appears that oral decongestants may work somewhat better on this problem.

Gastroschisis – Say What?

There have been a few studies which have analyzed a series of pregnancies that delivered children with a rare specific birth defect of the intestines and the abdominal wall called gastroschisis (gas-tro-SKEE-sis). One of the theories behind the cause of this specific birth defect is constricted blood vessels. Some of these studies identified a higher use of several of the decongestant drugs and other **drugs that affect blood vessels** when compared to patients who did not deliver babies with gastroschisis. Remember, a group of patients who deliver children with a specific birth defect is a population that probably has an underlying genetic risk for that birth defect. Therefore, this does not represent the general pregnant population.

ALL over-the-counter decongestant drugs constrict blood vessels; however, at this time we cannot identify those individuals who have a genetic predisposition for gastroschisis. An increase in gastroschisis has not been seen in any of the studies that analyzed the use of decongestant drugs in the general pregnant population. If you have a concern about this particular birth defect, then you should speak to your obstetrical caregiver before using any decongestant in the first trimester.

The Crux Of The Matter

This section may seem somewhat technical, but if you have one of the diseases or medical problems listed in the WARNINGS section near the beginning of the chapter, the following information will help to explain why the decongestant active ingredients are listed with warning labels attached to them.

Decongestants are a class of medications called sympathomimetic (sim-PATH-o-me-MET-ic) drugs. (I hope I didn't lose anyone after using the word sympathomimetic, but it's a great conversation stopper.) The sympathomimetic drugs can have an effect in many different places throughout the entire body. These drugs can be divided into **alpha agents** or **beta agents**, or ones that exhibit both alpha and beta activity.

A Little Bit Of History

Some of these active ingredients have been around for over a thousand years; however, this class of drugs was not really discovered until the late 1890s and early 1900s. The first sympathomimetic drug analyzed was **adrenaline** (a-DREN-al-in), a drug name frequently used on television or in stories that involve hospitals or doctors. The real name for adrenaline is

epinephrine (EP-uh-NEF-rin) and all decongestant drugs are related to adrenaline (epinephrine) in some way. The fact that sympathomimetic drugs have an alpha effect or beta effect was discovered around 1948 (about 50 years ago). During the 1950s and 1960s many studies were performed to determine what parts of the human body show an alpha effect or a beta effect or both.

Agents, Not Spies—In The Beginning Was Alpha

Alpha agents can affect or produce a reaction in the heart, the liver, the pancreas (which makes insulin among other things), and they can work on smooth muscles.

We Interrupt This Message For Muscle Types

Before I go any further, there are basically two types of muscles throughout our body: **skeletal** muscles and **smooth** muscles.

Skeletal muscles, found mostly around our bones or skeleton, help us move our arms and legs and fingers, and are also involved in the movement of our eyes and eyelids. Under a microscope, the muscle fibers appear to crisscross over each other.

Smooth muscles, on the other hand, are located in our body organs. They are found in our lungs, in the walls of our blood vessels, in the walls of our intestines, and **in the walls of the uterus**. Under a microscope the muscle fibers appear to head in one direction. The heart muscle is the only muscle that is slightly different than plain skeletal muscle or smooth muscle. (So I lied; there really are three types of muscle.)

Back To The Alpha Agents

Alpha agents cause the heart to beat faster and harder, cause the smooth muscles in blood vessels to contract or constrict (which could increase blood pressure), cause the pancreas to slow down the release of insulin (which could increase blood sugar), and cause the liver to break down and release stored up sugar into the bloodstream (which could also increase blood sugar).

Alpha agents can also make the smooth muscles in the intestines relax. As you can see, not all smooth muscles in the body react the same with alpha agents. Most smooth muscles contract or tighten in the presence of alpha agents, but some (like those found in the intestines) can relax. **For pregnant women**, alpha agents can cause the smooth muscles in the uterus to contract, which is important for you to know because this means they could cause uterine contractions.

Then Came Beta-1 And Beta-2

Beta agents can also have an effect or produce a reaction in the heart, liver, and smooth muscles. Beta agents may be described as primarily beta-1 agents and/or primarily beta-2 agents (it figures, doesn't it?). The beta-1 agents work mostly on the heart, while the beta-2 agents work mostly on the liver and smooth muscles. The beta-1 effect causes the heart to contract more strongly and usually causes the heart rate to increase or go faster.

The beta-2 effect on the liver causes stored up sugar to be broken down and released (which could increase blood sugar); however, it usually causes smooth muscles to relax. Therefore, beta-2 agents can cause the smooth muscles in the walls of blood vessels to relax (which may lower blood pressure), they can cause the smooth muscles in our lungs to relax (which allows air to flow in and out easier), and they can cause the smooth muscles in the uterus to relax. **For pregnant women** this means that beta-2 agents might slow down, stop or prevent uterine contractions.

To Recap

Remember, for those of you who are pregnant, alpha agents can cause blood vessels to constrict which makes it more difficult for blood to flow through and can increase blood pressure, whereas beta-2 agents will relax blood vessels which allows the blood to flow easier and may decrease blood pressure. In addition, alpha agents might make the uterus contract, whereas beta-2 agents might make the uterus relax. For easy reference, see Table 4 on page 263 for effects of alpha and beta drugs on various parts of the body.

From the discussion about alpha and beta effects on the heart, you can see that people with heart disease must be careful when they take drugs that have either an alpha or a beta effect because both can make the heart beat stronger and faster. People with high blood pressure should also be careful, because the alpha agent can increase blood pressure by constricting blood vessels. **Remember, any pregnant woman can develop toxemia** (high blood pressure or hypertension caused by the pregnancy). Furthermore, EVERY over-the-counter decongestant has the alpha effect (which is why they are effective), so all of them have the potential to cause hypertension. The de-congestants available in nasal sprays, nose drops, and nasal jellies are mostly alpha only agents, whereas the majority of oral decongestants are usually both alpha and beta in their action.

The Greek Letters And Diabetics

Diabetics must be careful because both alpha and beta agents can break down and release the liver's stored up sugar (glucose) which could significantly increase the amount of sugar in the bloodstream.

For those of you who might not remember, diabetes is a disease where a person has too much sugar in his or her bloodstream. In non-diabetic people, the pancreas produces the hormone insulin which lowers the level of blood sugar by facilitating the transport of glucose to the inside of our cells for use as energy. Almost everything we eat is eventually changed into glucose because the cells in our bodies use it for energy in order to function properly.

Without insulin, glucose cannot get inside our cells, and we end up with high blood sugar. People with diabetes cannot make insulin or do not make enough, so they have high blood sugar. Since alpha and beta agents can lead to a breakdown of stored-up sugar, this could increase blood sugar even more. In addition, alpha agents can also slow down the release of insulin from the pancreas, which would only make matters worse. Therefore, diabetics need to be aware of these issues before using any over-the-counter decongestant medication. People who do not have diabetes can usually handle these effects on blood sugar without difficulty, but diabetics may not. **Remember, any pregnant woman can develop gestational diabetes.**

The Silent Ones

At this point, it is important to recognize that many people are unaware they have high blood pressure or elevated blood sugar, and for this reason these diseases are sometimes called silent killers. Therefore, if you do not know whether or not you have high blood pressure or diabetes, it is recommended that you have regular physical checkups for your health and peace of mind.

Too Much Of A Good Thing

An overactive thyroid gland produces too much thyroid hormone and this can increase a person's heart rate and elevate blood pressure. This effect is similar to what could occur in the body when decongestant drugs are used. Therefore, these drugs may have an added effect on top of too much thyroid hormone. For this reason, people with an overactive thyroid gland should also be careful about using these medications.

The Eyes Have It Too

If you have an eye disease called narrow-angle glaucoma, using over-the-counter decongestant drugs may also cause problems. Because this condition involves elevated fluid pressure within the eyeball, you should speak with your ophthalmologist or healthcare provider before using a decongestant.

A Matter Of Occupation

Liver and kidney problems are included because the liver is the main organ that breaks down a drug once it is taken, and the kidneys usually remove it from the body. If the liver is not working well, it may take longer for the body to break down some of these drugs, and if the kidneys are not functioning properly it may take longer for the body to get rid of the drug. Therefore, the amount of drug taken or the frequency in which it is used may need adjustment.

A Place To Stay: Receptors

The decongestant drugs discussed in this chapter may have an alpha effect, a beta effect, or both. To expand a little bit, we have talked about how these agents or drugs may work on a particular part of the body. In reality, these body parts or organs have little places or spaces where these agents can attach themselves and cause their reaction to occur. These little spaces are called **receptors**. Some organs or body parts (like the heart, the liver, the blood vessels, and the uterus) have receptors for both alpha drugs and beta drugs.

Other organs may only have one type of receptor. A good example of this is our lungs. The smooth muscles inside the lungs essentially only have beta-2 receptors; therefore, if a drug has a beta-2 effect, it will cause the muscles in the lungs to relax and air will flow in and out easier. People with asthma have lungs that are constricted, so it is difficult for them to breathe (it is hard for the air to flow in and out). Scientists have developed drugs that primarily work on beta-2 receptors, and these are called beta-2 agonists or beta-2 drugs. Beta-2 drugs have also been used in the treatment of premature labor because they may slow down a woman's contractions.

As stated earlier, some drugs may have both alpha and beta effects. The best example of this is the drug called adrenaline (epinephrine). Adrenaline is very strong in both the alpha area and beta area. It works on the heart by making it beat harder, it constricts blood vessels through the alpha effect which increases blood pressure, and at the same time it can help a person who is having a severe asthma attack by relaxing the lungs through the beta effect.

Most of these sympathomimetic drugs are not pure alpha or pure beta in their actions. These drugs usually can affect both alpha and beta receptors, and the effects may be fairly equal between the two or may be exaggerated toward alpha or toward beta. Therefore, when we discuss the individual drugs in this chapter, you will notice words like primarily alpha or primarily beta, meaning that the drug has a larger influence in one of these areas.

Before using this medication, please read the following :
WARNINGS Section - page 88
DRUG INTERACTIONS Section - page 91
TWO SIDES OF SIDE EFFECTS Section - page 92

1. Oxymetazoline

Oxymetazoline (ox-ee-meh-TAZ-o-leen) is a decongestant drug found in nasal sprays, nose drops, or nasal jellies. If you read a label from an over-the-counter medication that has the word oxymetazoline (only), oxymetazoline hydrochloride, or oxymetazoline HCl, they all essentially mean the same thing. A common brand name (trade name) medication that contains this active ingredient is Afrin Nasal Spray. However, please remember that the active ingredients in a brand name product can change over time. Therefore, you still need to read the labels.

This medication works by constricting the blood vessels inside the nose and sinus area. To better understand this action, see the discussion on Nasal Sprays (page 96). Oxymetazoline is very similar to two other decongestants, xylometazoline and naphazoline. Basically, oxymetazoline is considered a long-acting decongestant drug when compared to other decongestants.

If You Are Pregnant

Oxymetazoline has not been proven to cause major birth defects in humans. One study[3] identified at least 255 pregnant women who used oxymetazoline in the first trimester, and no increase in major birth defects was seen over what was expected. Please read the section on gastroschisis found on page 98. (For statistical information on the number of pregnant women who took this drug in the first trimester compared to other decongestants, see Table 1 on page 260.) Animal studies during pregnancy on this particular drug were not found.

Based on the above information, this drug would be classified according to the pregnancy risk category as a C (see Chapter 4, How is Drug Safety Determined?).

No long-term effects that may show up later in life have been reported with the use of this drug during pregnancy.

Oxymetazoline is a fairly potent alpha agent (described in The Crux of the Matter, page 99). It has very little beta effect, if any. This means that oxymetazoline could constrict blood vessels throughout the body and raise one's blood pressure. One study that examined the use of this drug in a few healthy pregnant women (women who had no health problems in their pregnancy) found that using the recommended dose and frequency of this drug did not change blood flow in the uterus or the baby. Animal studies, however, on other alpha drugs have found a temporary decrease in blood flow through the uterus and, therefore, demonstrated that a constricting effect is possible. Again, **before you use** oxymetazoline or any other decongestant, you must find out if you have toxemia (high blood pressure during pregnancy) and this is discussed further in the WARNINGS section (pages 88-90).

Because oxymetazoline is primarily an alpha agent it could possibly lead to contractions of the uterus, but this question has not been studied to date. Information about the potential for this drug causing uterine contractions is based only upon how the muscles of the uterus react when exposed to an alpha drug. Therefore, if you have concerns or are at risk for premature labor, you should speak with your healthcare provider before using this medication.

Nasal Congestion of Pregnancy was discussed on page 96. Why this problem develops in some pregnancies is not fully understood. However, it is related to the fact that blood vessels become more dilated during pregnancy. Since the use of oxymetazoline is only recommended for three days because of the possibility of rebound congestion, it is not appropriate to use this drug for the treatment of nasal congestion of pregnancy. This is because nasal congestion of pregnancy may last for weeks or months.

Details About Oxymetazoline

- For dosing information, read the package material carefully because all drugs vary on the amount that can be used and the frequency of their use. However, nasal sprays, nose drops, and nasal jellies should not be used for more than three days.

- The onset of action (when you can expect some response) is within five to ten minutes of using the medicine.
- The duration of action (how long the effect might last) is six to seven hours or longer.
- The absorption (how much is taken into the bloodstream) varies from person to person. Also, the amount absorbed from the inside lining of the nose and throat is quite different from that absorbed in the intestines, if you swallow some. Remember, this is a nasal spray that often gets partly swallowed.
- The metabolism of the drug (how the body breaks down the drug) occurs in the liver; however, not all of the drug is metabolized.
- The elimination of the drug (how the body gets rid of it) is accomplished by the kidneys. The kidneys remove it from the body whether it is metabolized or not.
- The half-life of the drug (the amount of time it takes the body to remove half of the drug still circulating in the bloodstream) is about five to eight hours.

Further Issues

When talking about a stuffy nose caused by a cold or the flu, using this drug at the recommended dose and frequency for only one to three days would probably have little or no effect on a normal **uncomplicated** pregnancy. To use for a longer period of time could cause rebound congestion.

Many decongestants can stimulate the brain causing a feeling of being awake or nervous. An interesting finding with oxymetazoline is that it may also cause a depressed feeling in some people.

Breast-feeding

No thorough studies on breast-feeding and this drug have been reported. Some studies have looked at other alpha drugs which, if absorbed into the bloodstream, may be found in breast milk. However, in most cases, the amount of the alpha drugs found in breast milk was so small that any effect on the baby would most likely be unnoticed. This is especially true if recommended doses are used. In theory only, if larger than recommended doses were used, some irritability in the baby could be expected.

Before using this medication, please read the following :
WARNINGS Section - page 88
DRUG INTERACTIONS Section - page 91
TWO SIDES OF SIDE EFFECTS Section - page 92

2. Xylometazoline

Xylometazoline (ZI-low-meh-TAZ-o-leen) is another decongestant drug that is found in nasal sprays, nose drops, or nasal jellies. If you read a label from an over-the-counter medication that has the word xylometazoline (only), xylometazoline hydrochloride, or xylometazoline HCl, they all essentially mean the same thing. A common brand name (trade name) medication that contains this active ingredient is Otrivin Nasal Spray. However, please remember that the active ingredients in a brand name product can change over time. Therefore, you still need to read the labels.

Much of the information in this section is similar to that of oxymetazoline because the two drugs are so similar. Therefore, at times you may be referred back to the oxymetazoline section for some of the issues involving this drug.

This medication works by constricting the blood vessels inside the nose and sinus area. To better understand this action, see the discussion on Nasal Sprays (page 96). Xylometazoline is very similar to two other decongestants, oxymetazoline and naphazoline. Xylometazoline is considered a long-acting decongestant drug when compared to other decongestants.

If You Are Pregnant

Xylometazoline has not been proven to cause major birth defects in humans. One study[3] identified 461 pregnant women who used xylometazoline in the first trimester, and no increase in major birth defects was seen over what was expected. Please read the section on gastroschisis found on page 98. (For statistical information on the number of pregnant women who took this drug in the first trimester compared to other decongestants, see Table 1 on page 260.) Animal studies during pregnancy on this particular drug were not found.

Based on the above information, this drug would be classified according to the pregnancy risk category as a C (see Chapter 4, How is Drug Safety Determined?).

No long-term effects that may show up later in life have been reported with the use of this drug during pregnancy.

Xylometazoline (like oxymetazoline) is a fairly potent alpha agent (described in The Crux of the Matter, page 99). It has very little beta effect, if any. This means that xylometazoline could constrict blood vessels throughout the body, could raise one's blood pressure, might cause uterine contractions, and has the same precautions for use in the treatment of Nasal Congestion of Pregnancy (see pages 107-108 under Oxymetazoline). Again, **before you use** xylometazoline or any other decongestant, you must find out if you have toxemia (high blood pressure during pregnancy) and this is discussed further in the WARNINGS section (pages 88-90).

Details About Xylometazoline

- For dosing information, read the package material carefully because all drugs vary on the amount that can be used and the frequency of their use. However, nasal sprays, nose drops, and nasal jellies should not be used for more than three days.
- The onset of action (when you can expect some response) is within five to ten minutes of using the medicine.
- The duration of action (how long the effect might last) is five to six hours or longer.
- The absorption (how much is taken into the bloodstream) varies from person to person. Also, the amount absorbed from the inside lining of the nose and throat is quite different from that absorbed in the intestines, if you swallow some. Remember, this is a nasal spray that often gets partly swallowed.
- The metabolism of the drug (how the body breaks down the drug) occurs in the liver; however, not all of the drug is metabolized.
- The elimination of the drug (how the body gets rid of it) is accomplished by the kidneys. The kidneys remove it from the body whether it is metabolized or not.
- The half-life of the drug (the amount of time it takes the body to remove half of the drug still circulating in the bloodstream) is about five to eight hours.

Further Issues

When talking about a stuffy nose caused by a cold or the flu, using this drug at the recommended dose and frequency for only one to three days would probably have little or no effect on a normal **uncomplicated** pregnancy. To use for a longer period of time could cause rebound congestion.

Many decongestants can stimulate the brain causing a feeling of being awake or nervous. An interesting finding with xylometazoline is that it may also cause a depressed feeling in some people.

Breast-feeding

No thorough studies on breast-feeding and this drug have been reported. Some studies have looked at other alpha drugs which, if absorbed into the bloodstream, may be found in breast milk. However, in most cases, the amount of the alpha drugs found in breast milk was so small that any effect on the baby would most likely be unnoticed. This is especially true if recommended doses are used. In theory only, if larger than recommended doses were used, some irritability in the baby could be expected.

Before using this medication, please read the following :
WARNINGS Section - page 88
DRUG INTERACTIONS Section - page 91
TWO SIDES OF SIDE EFFECTS Section - page 92

3. Naphazoline

Naphazoline (na-FAZ-o-leen) is another decongestant drug that is found in nasal sprays, nose drops, or nasal jellies. If you read a label from an over-the-counter medication that has the word naphazoline (only), naphazoline hydrochloride, or naphazoline HCl, they all essentially mean the same thing.

A common brand name (trade name) medication that contains this active ingredient is Privine Nasal Spray. However, please remember that the active ingredients in a brand name product can change over time. Therefore, you still need to read the labels.

Much of the information in this section is similar to that of oxymetazoline because they are so similar. Therefore, at times you may be referred back to the oxymetazoline section for some of the issues involving this drug.

This medication works by constricting the blood vessels inside the nose and sinus area. To better understand this action, see the discussion on Nasal Sprays (page 96). Naphazoline is very similar to two other decongestants, oxymetazoline and xylometazoline. Naphazoline is considered a short-acting decongestant drug when compared to other decongestants.

If You Are Pregnant

Naphazoline has not been proven to cause major birth defects in humans. In one study[1], only 20 patients with first trimester exposure to this drug were identified, and no increase in major birth defects was seen over what was expected. Please read the section on gastroschisis found on page 98. (For statistical information on the number of pregnant women who took this drug in the first trimester compared to other decongestants, see Table 1 on page 260.) Animal studies during pregnancy on this particular drug were not found.

Based on the above information, this drug would be classified according to the pregnancy risk category as a C (see Chapter 4, How is Drug Safety Determined?).

No long-term effects that may show up later in life have been reported with the use of this drug during pregnancy.

Naphazoline (like oxymetazoline) is a fairly potent alpha agent (described in The Crux of the Matter, page 99). It has very little beta effect, if any. This means that naphazoline could constrict blood vessels throughout the body, could raise one's blood pressure, might cause uterine contractions, and has the same precautions for use in the treatment of Nasal Congestion of Pregnancy (see pages 107-108 under Oxymetazoline). Again, **before you use** naphazoline or any other decongestant, you must find out if you have toxemia (high blood pressure during pregnancy) and this is discussed further in the WARNINGS section (pages 88-90).

Details About Naphazoline

- For dosing information, read the package material carefully because all drugs vary on the amount that can be used and the frequency of their use. However, nasal sprays, nose drops, and nasal jellies should not be used for more than three days.

- The onset of action (when you can expect some response) is within five to ten minutes of using the medicine.

- The duration of action (how long the effect might last) is two to six hours.

- The absorption (how much is taken into the bloodstream) varies from person to person. Also, the amount absorbed from the inside lining of the nose and throat is quite different from that absorbed in the intestines, if you swallow some. Remember, this is a nasal spray that often gets partly swallowed.

- The metabolism of the drug (how the body breaks down the drug) occurs in the liver; however, not all of the drug is metabolized.
- The elimination of the drug (how the body gets rid of it) is accomplished by the kidneys. The kidneys remove it from the body whether it is metabolized or not.
- The half-life of the drug (the amount of time it takes the body to remove half of the drug still circulating in the bloodstream) is about three to six hours.

Further Issues

When talking about a stuffy nose caused by a cold or the flu, using this drug at the recommended dose and frequency for only one to three days would probably have little or no effect on a normal **uncomplicated** pregnancy. To use for a longer period of time could cause rebound congestion.

Many decongestants can stimulate the brain causing a feeling of being awake or nervous. An interesting finding with naphazoline is that it may also cause a depressed feeling in some people.

Breast-feeding

No thorough studies on breast-feeding and this drug have been reported. Some studies have looked at other alpha drugs which, if absorbed into the bloodstream, may be found in breast milk. However, in most cases, the amount of the alpha drugs found in breast milk was so small that any effect on the baby would most likely be unnoticed. This is especially true if recommended doses are used. In theory only, if larger than recommended doses were used, some irritability in the baby could be expected.

Before using this medication, please read the following :
WARNINGS Section - page 88
DRUG INTERACTIONS Section - page 91
TWO SIDES OF SIDE EFFECTS Section - page 92

4. Propylhexedrine

Propylhexedrine (pro-pull-HEX-id-dreen) is another decongestant drug that is found in nasal sprays, nose drops, or nasal jellies. A common brand name (trade name) medication that contains this active ingredient is Benzedrex. However, please remember that the active ingredients in a brand name product can change over time. Therefore, you still need to read the labels.

Much of the information in this section is similar to that of oxymetazoline because they are so similar. Therefore, at times you may be referred back to the oxymetazoline section for some of the issues involving this drug.

Propylhexedrine works by constricting the blood vessels inside the nose and sinus area. To better understand this action, see the discussion on Nasal Sprays (page 96). Propylhexedrine is considered a short-acting decongestant drug when compared to other decongestants.

If You Are Pregnant

Propylhexedrine has not been proven to cause major birth defects in humans. One study[1] only identified five patients with first trimester exposure to this drug, but exact details regarding outcome were not supplied. Please read the section on gastroschisis found on page 98. (For statistical information on the number of pregnant women who took this drug in the first trimester compared to other decongestants, see Table 1 on page 260.) Animal studies during pregnancy on this particular drug were not found.

Based on the above information, this drug would be classified according to the pregnancy risk category as a C (see Chapter 4, How is Drug Safety Determined?).

No long-term effects that may show up later in life have been reported with the use of this drug during pregnancy.

Propylhexedrine is a fairly potent alpha agent (described in The Crux of the Matter, page 99). It has very little beta effect, if any. This means that propylhexedrine could constrict blood vessels throughout the body, could raise one's blood pressure, might cause uterine contractions, and has the same precautions for use in the treatment of Nasal Congestion of Pregnancy (see pages 107-108 under Oxymetazoline). Again, **before you use** propylhexedrine or any other decongestant, you must find out if you have toxemia (high blood pressure during pregnancy), and this is discussed further in the WARNINGS section (pages 88-90).

Details About Propylhexedrine

- For dosing information, read the package material carefully because all drugs vary on the amount that can be used and the frequency of their use. However, nasal sprays, nose drops, and nasal jellies should not be used for more than three days.

- The onset of action (when you can expect some response) is within five to ten minutes of using the medicine.

- The duration of action (how long the effect might last) is about two hours.

- The absorption (how much is taken into the bloodstream) varies from person to person. Also, the amount absorbed from the inside lining of the nose and throat is quite different from that absorbed in the intestines, if you swallow some. Remember, this is a nasal spray that often gets partly swallowed.

- The metabolism of the drug (how the body breaks down the drug) occurs in the liver.
- The elimination of the drug (how the body gets rid of it) is accomplished by the kidneys. The kidneys remove it from the body whether it is metabolized or not.
- The half-life of the drug (the amount of time it takes the body to remove half of the drug still circulating in the bloodstream) is about three to four hours.

Further Issues

When talking about a stuffy nose caused by a cold or the flu, using this drug at the recommended dose and frequency for only one to three days would probably have little or no effect on a normal **uncomplicated** pregnancy. To use for a longer period of time could cause rebound congestion.

Breast-feeding

No thorough studies on breast-feeding and this drug have been reported. Some studies have looked at other alpha drugs which, if absorbed into the bloodstream, may be found in breast milk. However, in most cases, the amount of the alpha drugs found in breast milk was so small that any effect on the baby would most likely be unnoticed. This is especially true if recommended doses are used. In theory only, if larger than recommended doses were used, some irritability in the baby could be expected.

Before using this medication, please read the following :
WARNINGS Section - page 88
DRUG INTERACTIONS Section - page 91
TWO SIDES OF SIDE EFFECTS Section - page 92

5. Phenylephrine

Phenylephrine (fen-ILL-eff-rin) is a decongestant drug primarily found in nasal sprays, nose drops, or nasal jellies AND is also contained within some of the cold remedies that are taken orally in the form of pills, tablets, or capsules. If you read a label from an over-the-counter medication that has the word phenylephrine (only), phenylephrine hydrochloride, phenylephrine HCl, or phenylephrine bitartrate, they all essentially mean the same thing. Because this drug also comes in pill form, a full description is given even though there is duplicated information with that of oxymetazoline in some areas.

A common brand name (trade name) medication that contains this active ingredient is Neo-Synephrine. However, please remember that the active ingredients in a brand name product can change over time. Therefore, you still need to read the labels.

This medication works by constricting the blood vessels inside the nose and sinus area. To better understand this action, see the discussion on Nasal Sprays (page 96). Phenylephrine, as a nasal spray, nose drops, or nasal jelly, is considered a short-acting decongestant drug when compared to other decongestants.

If You Are Pregnant

Phenylephrine has not been proven to cause major birth defects in humans. From two studies[1,3], a total of at least 1,650 pregnant women were identified who used phenylephrine in the first trimester, and no increase in major birth defects was seen over what was expected. In one of these studies[1], there were 4,194 women who used this drug at some time in their pregnancy (all three trimesters), and no increase in major birth defects was identified. Please read the section on gastroschisis found on page 98. (For statistical information on the number of pregnant women who took this drug in the first trimester compared to other decongestants, see Table 1 on page 260.) Animal studies during pregnancy on this particular drug were not found.

Despite the above information, this drug would still be classified according to the pregnancy risk category as a C (see Chapter 4, How is Drug Safety Determined?).

No long-term effects that may show up later in life have been reported with the use of this drug during pregnancy.

Phenylephrine is a fairly potent alpha agent (described in The Crux of the Matter, page 99). It has very little beta effect, if any. This means that phenylephrine could constrict blood vessels throughout the body and raise one's blood pressure. There are animal studies on phenylephrine and other alpha drugs that found a temporary decrease in blood flow through the uterus and, therefore, demonstrated that a constricting effect is possible. Again, **before you use** phenylephrine or any other decongestant, you must find out if you have toxemia (high blood pressure during pregnancy) and this is discussed further in the WARNINGS section (pages 88-90).

Because phenylephrine is primarily an alpha agent it could possibly lead to contractions of the uterus. This question has not been thoroughly studied to date. Information about the potential for this drug causing uterine contractions is based only upon how the muscles of the uterus react when exposed to an alpha drug. Therefore, if you have concerns or are at risk for premature labor, you should speak with your healthcare provider before using this medication.

Nasal Congestion of Pregnancy was discussed on page 96. Why this problem develops in some pregnancies is not fully understood. However, it is related to the fact that blood vessels become more dilated during pregnancy. Since the use of phenylephrine (as a nasal spray) is only recommended for three days because of the possibility of rebound congestion, it is not appropriate to use this drug for the treatment of nasal congestion of pregnancy. This is because nasal congestion of pregnancy may last for weeks or months.

When phenylephrine is used in pill form, the time of use can be extended up to seven to ten days because rebound congestion is not considered a problem. Phenylephrine, however, is not generally found exclusively by itself in pill form but is usually combined with other drugs found in this book.

Details About Phenylephrine

- For dosing information, read the package material carefully because all drugs vary on the amount that can be used and the frequency of their use. However, nasal sprays, nose drops, and nasal jellies should not be used for more than three days.

- The onset of action (when you can expect some response) is within five to ten minutes of using the nasal spray medication, or within 15 to 30 minutes when taken as pills.

- The duration of action (how long the effect might last) is three to six hours.

- The absorption (how much is taken into the bloodstream) varies from person to person. Also, the amount absorbed from the inside lining of the nose and throat is quite different from that absorbed in the intestines, if you swallow some. Remember, as a nasal spray, some of the liquid gets partly swallowed. This drug also comes in pill form. Compared to the other pill decongestants, this one is absorbed the least; however, the drug is still found in the bloodstream after usage.

- The metabolism of the drug (how the body breaks down the drug) occurs in the liver; however, some of the drug is metabolized in the intestines before it is absorbed.

- The elimination of the drug (how the body gets rid of it) is accomplished by the kidneys. The kidneys remove it from the body whether it is metabolized or not.

- The half-life of the drug (the amount of time it takes the body to remove half of the drug still circulating in the bloodstream) is about two to three hours.

Further Issues

When talking about a stuffy nose caused by a cold or the flu, using this drug at the recommended dose and frequency would probably have little or no effect on a normal **uncomplicated** pregnancy. Using phenylephrine as a nasal spray for longer than three days could cause rebound congestion.

Phenylephrine is also used by some hospitals in the intensive care unit where the drug is injected into a vein to increase a person's blood pressure (for those people who have critically low blood pressure). Therefore, it is well known that phenylephrine in the bloodstream can increase blood pressure.

Again, this effect on blood pressure is very important to understand, especially if you already have hypertension or you have toxemia while pregnant.

Breast-feeding

No thorough studies on breast-feeding and this drug have been reported. Some studies have looked at other alpha drugs which, if absorbed into the bloodstream, may be found in breast milk. However, in most cases, the amount of the alpha drugs found in breast milk was so small that any effect on the baby would most likely be unnoticed. This is especially true for phenylephrine due to its poor absorption from the intestines in general. If the drug were found in breast milk, the baby would also probably absorb very little from its own intestines. In theory only, if larger than recommended doses were used, some irritability in the baby could be expected.

Before using this medication, please read the following :
WARNINGS Section - page 88
DRUG INTERACTIONS Section - page 91
TWO SIDES OF SIDE EFFECTS Section - page 92

6. *Pseudoephedrine*

Pseudoephedrine (soo-doe-ef-FED-rin) is a decongestant drug primarily found in cold remedies that are taken orally in the form of pills, tablets or capsules. If you read a label from an over-the-counter medication that has the word pseudoephedrine (only), pseudoephedrine hydrochloride, pseudoephedrine HCl, or pseudoephedrine sulfate, they all essentially mean the same thing.

A common brand name (trade name) medication that contains this active ingredient is Sudafed; however, numerous OTC products contain pseudoephedrine. Please remember that the active ingredients in a brand name product can change over time. Therefore, you still need to read the labels.

This medication works by constricting the blood vessels inside the nose and sinus area. To better understand this action, see the discussion on Nasal Sprays (page 96), even though this drug only comes in pill form. In addition, the first five drugs of this chapter were primarily alpha agents. Pseudoephedrine has **both alpha and beta effects**. Pseudoephedrine is marketed as regular-acting pills or long-acting pills (usually given the name sustained release or extended release tablets).

If You Are Pregnant

Pseudoephedrine has not been proven to cause major birth defects in humans. From three large studies[1-3], a total of 2,509 pregnant women were identified who used pseudoephedrine in the first trimester, and no increase in major birth defects was seen over what was expected. From two of these studies[1,2], there were 2,113 women who used this drug at some time in their pregnancy (all three trimesters), and no increase in major birth defects was identified. Please read the section on gastroschisis found on page 98. (For statistical information on the number of pregnant women who took this drug in the first trimester compared to other decongestants, see Table 1 on page 260.) This drug has also been studied in pregnant animals that were given doses larger than those recommended for humans, and no harm was identified.

Despite the above information, this drug would still be classified according to the pregnancy risk category as a C (see Chapter 4, How is Drug Safety Determined?).

No long-term effects that may show up later in life have been reported with the use of this drug during pregnancy.

Pseudoephedrine is a drug that has both an alpha and a beta effect (described in The Crux of the Matter, page 99). Because it has an alpha effect, it might constrict blood vessels throughout the body, which then could increase blood pressure. Again, **before you use** pseudoephedrine or any other decongestant, you must find out if you have toxemia (high blood pressure during pregnancy) and this is discussed further in the WARNINGS section (pages 88-90).

The fact that pseudoephedrine has an alpha effect also means that it could lead to contractions in the uterus. HOWEVER, since this drug also has a **beta effect**, this would tend to relax the uterus. The question of uterine contractions and pseudoephedrine use has not yet been studied. However, based on the fact that muscles of the uterus relax when exposed to beta drugs, there probably would be either no effect on the uterus or the uterus would tend to relax if exposed to pseudoephedrine.

Nasal Congestion of Pregnancy was discussed on page 96. Decongestants that come in pill form can be used for a longer period of time (seven to ten days) when compared to the nasal sprays, nose drops, or nasal jellies. The use of decongestant pills in treating nasal congestion of pregnancy is also in question because this problem usually lasts for more than a week. Therefore, this should be discussed with your healthcare provider.

Details About Pseudoephedrine

- For dosing information, read the package material carefully because all drugs vary on the amount that can be used and the frequency of their use.
- The onset of action (when you can expect some response) is usually within 15 to 30 minutes of taking the medicine.
- The duration of action (how long the effect might last) is about four hours for the regular pills and up to 8 to 12 hours for the sustained or extended release pills.
- The absorption (how much is taken into the bloodstream) occurs in the intestines, and most of an oral dose is absorbed.
- The metabolism of the drug (how the body breaks down the drug) occurs in the liver. However, only about 10 to 30 percent is broken down. The rest of the drug remains unchanged in the bloodstream until it is eliminated.
- The elimination of the drug (how the body gets rid of it) is accomplished by the kidneys. The kidneys remove it from the body whether it is metabolized or not.
- The half-life of the drug (the amount of time it takes the body to remove half of the drug still circulating in the bloodstream) is about 9 to 16 hours. The ability of the kidneys to eliminate this drug from the body is somewhat dependent upon the pH of the urine. If the urine has a low pH (more acidic) the drug is removed more quickly. If the urine pH is normal, the half-life removal is about 9 to 16 hours. If the urine has a high pH (more alkaline), it takes longer for the body to remove the drug (a half-life that could be up to two full days in length with a urine pH over 7.5).

Further Issues

When talking about a stuffy nose caused by a cold or the flu, using this drug at the recommended dose and frequency would probably have little or no effect on a normal **uncomplicated** pregnancy.

Another important issue that pertains primarily to this drug is that the pills, especially extended-release pills, **should never be crushed** prior to their use. This might result in a greater amount of drug being absorbed too quickly into the bloodstream increasing the chance for affecting blood pressure. Also, the use of **antacids may increase** the amount of drug absorbed from the intestines. Pregnant women often suffer from heartburn, and the use of antacids is common. If you are using an antacid, you may want to start with a lower dose of this medication, especially if you are pregnant.

Breast-feeding

Very little information is found involving this drug and breast-feeding. One small study examined the amount of pseudoephedrine in breast milk in a few women who were using the drug as prescribed and found the quantity to be very small. More than likely this amount would not have an effect on a nursing child. In theory only, if larger than recommended doses were taken, some irritability in the baby might be expected. The American Academy of Pediatrics states that using pseudoephedrine is compatible with or acceptable while breast-feeding.

Before using this medication, please read the following :
WARNINGS Section - page 88
DRUG INTERACTIONS Section - page 91
TWO SIDES OF SIDE EFFECTS Section - page 92

7. Phenylpropanolamine

Phenylpropanolamine (fen-ill-PRO-pa-NOLE-a-meen) is a decongestant drug primarily found in cold remedies that are taken orally in the form of pills, tablets, or capsules. If you read a label from an over-the-counter medication that has the word phenylpropanolamine (only), phenylpropanolamine hydrochloride, phenylpropanolamine HCl, or phenylpropanolamine bitartrate, they all essentially mean the same thing.

A common brand name (trade name) medication that contains this active ingredient is Contac; however, numerous OTC products contain phenylpropanolamine. Please remember that the active ingredients in a brand name product can change over time. Therefore, you still need to read the labels.

This medication works by constricting the blood vessels inside the nose and sinus area. To better understand this action, see the discussion on Nasal Sprays (page 96), even though this drug only comes in pill form. This drug is like pseudoephedrine and has **both alpha and beta** effects and is different from drugs 1 through 5 described in this chapter. Phenylpropanolamine is marketed as regular-acting pills or long-acting pills (usually given the name sustained release or extended release tablets).

If You Are Pregnant

Phenylpropanolamine has not been proven to cause major birth defects in humans. From two studies[1,2], a total of at least 1,080 pregnant women were identified who used phenylpropanolamine in the first trimester, and no increase in major birth defects was seen over what was expected. In one of these studies[1], there were 2,489 women who used this drug at some time in their pregnancy (all three trimesters), and no increase in major birth defects was identified. Please read the section on gastroschisis found on page 98. (For statistical information on the number of pregnant women who took this drug in the first trimester compared to other decongestants, see Table 1 on page 260.) This drug has also been studied in pregnant animals that were given doses larger than those recommended for humans and no harm was identified.

Despite the above information, this drug would still be classified according to the pregnancy risk category as a C (see Chapter 4, How is Drug Safety Determined?).

No long-term effects that may show up later in life have been reported with the use of this drug during pregnancy.

Phenylpropanolamine is a drug that has both an alpha and a beta effect (described in The Crux of the Matter, page 99). Because it has an alpha effect, it might constrict blood vessels throughout the body, which then could increase blood pressure. Again, **before you use** phenylpropanolamine or any other decongestant, you must find out if you have toxemia (high blood pressure during pregnancy) and this is discussed further in the WARNINGS section (pages 88-90).

The fact that phenylpropanolamine has an alpha effect also means that it could lead to contractions in the uterus. HOWEVER, since this drug also has a **beta effect**, this would tend to relax the uterus. The question of uterine contractions and phenylpropanolamine has not yet been studied. However, based on the fact that muscles of the uterus relax when exposed to beta drugs, there probably would be either no effect on the uterus or the uterus would tend to relax if exposed to this drug.

Nasal Congestion of Pregnancy was discussed on page 96. Decongestants that come in pill form can be used for a longer period of time (seven to ten days) when compared to the nasal sprays, nose drops, or nasal jellies. The use of decongestant pills in treating nasal congestion of pregnancy is also in question because this problem usually lasts for more than a week. Therefore, this should be discussed with your healthcare provider.

Details About Phenylpropanolamine

- For dosing information, read the package material carefully because all drugs vary on the amount that can be used and the frequency of their use.

- The onset of action (when you can expect some response) is usually within 30 minutes of taking the medicine.

- The duration of action (how long the effect might last) is about four hours for the regular pills and up to 8 to 12 hours for the sustained or extended release pills.

- The absorption (how much is taken into the bloodstream) occurs in the intestines, with about 90 percent of an oral dose being absorbed.

- The metabolism of the drug (how the body breaks down the drug) occurs in the liver; however, only a small amount is broken down. The rest of the drug remains unchanged in the bloodstream until it is eliminated.

- The elimination of the drug (how the body gets rid of it) is accomplished by the kidneys. The kidneys remove it from the body whether it is metabolized or not.

- The half-life of the drug (the amount of time it takes the body to remove half of the drug still circulating in the bloodstream) is about five to seven hours. The ability of the kidneys to eliminate this drug from the body is also somewhat dependent upon the pH of the urine, but this effect is less than what is seen with pseudoephedrine (see page 127 under Pseudoephedrine).

Further Issues

When talking about a stuffy nose caused by a cold or the flu, using this drug at the recommended dose and frequency would probably have little or no effect on a normal **uncomplicated** pregnancy.

Another important issue that pertains primarily to this drug is that the pills, especially extended-release pills, **should never be crushed** prior to their use. This might result in a greater amount of drug being absorbed too quickly into the bloodstream increasing the chance for affecting blood pressure. Also, the use of **antacids may increase** the amount of drug absorbed from the intestines. Pregnant women often suffer from heartburn, and the use of antacids is common. If you are using an antacid, you may want to start with a smaller amount of this medication, especially if you are pregnant.

Breast-feeding

No thorough studies on breast-feeding and this drug have been reported. One small study was performed on a similar decongestant (pseudoephedrine) and the amount of drug found in breast milk was very small. In theory only, if larger than recommended doses were taken, some irritability in the baby might be expected.

Before using this medication, please read the following :
WARNINGS Section - page 88
DRUG INTERACTIONS Section - page 91
TWO SIDES OF SIDE EFFECTS Section - page 92

8. Levmetamfetamine

Levmetamfetamine (LEV-met-am-FET-uh-meen) is a decongestant drug found in a nasal spray inhaler. For years this active ingredient was called L-desoxyephedrine (EL-des-ox-ee-ef-FED-drin). In 1998 the U.S. Food and Drug Administration in conjunction with the United States Pharmacopoeia (USP) decided to change the name because the base drug was more similar to amphetamines (am-FET-uh-meens). A common brand name (trade name) medication that contains this active ingredient is Vicks Vapor Inhaler. However, please remember that the active ingredients in a brand name product can change over time. Therefore, you still need to read the labels.

Although the base drug is considered an amphetamine, it has very little (if any) stimulating effects on the brain like the amphetamines that are often abused. This drug is the mirror image of dextro-methamphetamine. At this point, I need to explain mirror image drugs. Get up from where you are and stand in front of a mirror. Now lift up your right hand and wave it. I know this sounds dumb, but the person in the mirror (hopefully you) is waving back with what seems to be the left hand. This is because the person in the mirror is your exact opposite.

Believe it or not, drugs also have exact opposites. In the chemistry of drugs, to explain one drug in relationship to its mirror image we sometimes say that the drugs are left or right. In medical or chemical terminology we often use the words **levo for left** and **dextro for right**, meaning they are exact opposites of each other (left-handed and right-handed). Therefore, if I put levmetamfetamine in front of a mirror, the drug staring back from the mirror would be dextro-methamphetamine.

Another **very important fact** is that mirror image drugs do not always work the same. Again, it is probably easier to explain this with an example.

Let's say there is a pain medicine called "levo-pain" so its mirror image is "dextro-pain." "Levo-pain" may work very well in taking away your pain. However, "dextro-pain" could be stronger, could be the same, could be weaker, or might have no action whatsoever when compared to "levo-pain."

Levmetamfetamine constricts blood vessels (which gives it decongestant properties), and in large amounts could increase blood pressure. However, it does not stimulate the brain causing euphoria or an elevation in mood (like dextromethamphetamine). Despite the fact that the base drug is an amphetamine (and is slightly different from the other decongestants), it still has the same warnings, drug interactions, and side effects of the other decongestants in this chapter.

This medication only comes in the form of a nasal spray and is considered a short-acting decongestant drug when compared to other nasal spray decongestants.

If You Are Pregnant

Levmetamfetamine has not been proven to cause major birth defects in humans. This specific drug has not been directly studied in human pregnancy. However, the amphetamine class of drugs has had numerous evaluations published. From one large study[1], a total of 671 pregnant women were identified who used amphetamines (amphetamine, dextroamphetamine and dextro-methamphetamine) in the first trimester, and no increase in major birth defects was seen over what was expected. In this same study, there were 1,898 women who used amphetamines at some time in their pregnancy (all three trimesters), and no increase in major birth defects was identified. Please read the section on gastroschisis found on page 98. (For statistical information on the number of pregnant women who took this drug in the first trimester compared to other decongestants, see Table 1 on page 260.) Animal studies during pregnancy on amphetamines have been performed and an **increase** in birth defects of the heart was seen when doses **200 times larger** than a human dose were given.

Numerous studies have analyzed a group of pregnant women who delivered children with heart defects (and other anomalies), and the number of women who used amphetamines was higher when compared to pregnancies that did not deliver children with heart defects. However, when many of these studies examined family histories, a higher rate of heart anomalies and birth defects was dectected, suggesting an underlying genetic risk. Most studies that have analyzed the amphetamine class of drugs in the random pregnant population have not found an increase in major birth defects.

Amphetamine drugs can rapidly cross the placenta and in large amounts can increase the blood pressure of the baby. There are also reports of smaller birth weights and babies going through withdrawal when mothers abused amphetamines during pregnancy. All of these studies have primary involved the dextro types of amphetamines, **not the levo forms**.

Because of the above conflicting information, this drug would be classified according to the pregnancy risk category as a C (see Chapter 4, How is Drug Safety Determined?). If amphetamines were used for their stimulation and euphoric effects, then they would be classified as a category X drug for pregnancy.

No long-term effects that may show up later in life have been reported with the use of levmetamfetamine during pregnancy.

Levmetamfetamine is a fairly potent alpha agent (described in The Crux of the Matter, page 99). It has very little beta effect, if any. This means that levmetamfetamine could constrict blood vessels throughout the body, could raise one's blood pressure, might cause uterine contractions, and has the same precautions for use in the treatment of Nasal Congestion of Pregnancy (see pages 107-108 under Oxymetazoline). Again, **before you use** levmetamfetamine or any other decongestant, you must find out if you have toxemia (high blood pressure during pregnancy) and this is discussed further in the WARNINGS section (pages 88-90).

Details About Levmetamfetamine

- For dosing information, read the package material carefully because all drugs vary on the amount that can be used and the frequency of their use. However, nasal sprays, nose drops, and nasal jellies should not be used for more than three days.
- The onset of action (when you can expect some response) is within five to ten minutes of using the medicine.
- The duration of action (how long the effect might last) is about two hours.
- The absorption (how much is taken into the bloodstream) varies from person to person. The amount absorbed from the intestines is quite high and, remember, some of the nasal spray liquid ends up being swallowed.
- The metabolism of the drug (how the body breaks down the drug) occurs in the liver. Some of the drug remains unchanged in the bloodstream until it is eliminated.
- The elimination of the drug (how the body gets rid of it) is accomplished by the kidneys. The kidneys remove it from the body whether it is metabolized or not.
- The half-life of the drug (the amount of time it takes the body to remove half of the drug still circulating in the bloodstream) is about three to six hours.

Further Issues

When talking about a stuffy nose caused by a cold or the flu, using this drug at the recommended dose and frequency for only one to three days would probably have little or no effect on a normal **uncomplicated** pregnancy. To use for a longer period of time could cause rebound congestion.

The amount of levmetamfetamine in an **entire inhaler** is only 50 milligrams. This is another important issue because adult prescription doses of amphetamine for treating obesity and narcolepsy (a condition where a person may suddenly fall asleep for no apparent reason) are in the range of 10 to 30 milligrams a day. These prescription medications primarily contain the dextro products. Levmetamfetamine is **20 to 30 times less potent** for causing euphoria and stimulation of the brain when compared to the dextro-amphetamines. Therefore, addiction and abuse are very unlikely; however, as with all decongestants, dependence can develop in some individuals.

Breast-feeding

No thorough studies on breast-feeding and this drug have been reported. Amphetamines as a class of drugs can be found in breast milk and have been found in the urine of nursing infants. No problems were reported; however, the American Academy of Pediatrics considers breast-feeding while taking amphetamines contraindicated.

8. Antihistamines

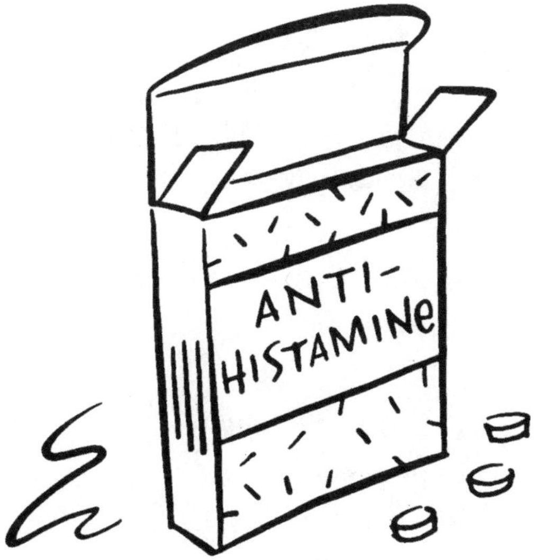

The antihistamines are a group or class of drugs that temporarily alleviate the symptoms of a runny nose and watery eyes. Some of the FDA recommended ways of describing what these medications may do are: temporarily relieves, decreases, alleviates, or helps dry up a runny nose. Also, they may temporarily alleviate, decrease, or reduce sneezing, and/or the symptoms of an itchy nose, itchy throat, itchy eyes, or watery eyes. From those descriptions, you can see that their use is geared more toward treating allergies than treating the effects of the common cold or the flu. However, many over-the-counter cold or flu products contain antihistamines.

What does the word antihistamine mean? Well, it is a drug that is **anti** or **against** something called **histamine**, but this will be explained later in the section called Stepping Back Into History. For now, please read the next few sections before you turn to the actual drugs.

WARNINGS

Before using any OTC antihistamine medication, persons with any of the following health problems should talk to their healthcare provider first.

- Heart disease
- High blood pressure
- Diabetes
- Respiratory problems (like asthma or chronic bronchitis)
- Narrow-angle glaucoma
- Difficulty urinating
- Stomach or intestinal ulcers
- Overactive thyroid gland
- Kidney problems
- Liver problems

Reasons for these warnings are explained in detail in the section called The Crux of the Matter. If you have one or more of the above medical conditions, using an antihistamine could cause problems. Also, a major caution associated with these drugs is that they can make a person sleepy or tired and, therefore, should not be used while driving or operating equipment.

Drug Interactions

Drug interactions means that if a person is using one medication and then decides to take an antihistamine, the two drugs might react with each other and cause problems. If you are taking another over-the-counter medicine or a drug prescribed by a doctor, and then you decide to take an antihistamine, be sure there is no conflict between the two medications. In addition, **you should not drink alcohol** while using antihistamines. The list below contains many of the drug categories that you should be familiar with because they might react with antihistamines.

- **Drugs that may make you tired**

This includes sleeping pills, tranquilizers, pain medicines, drugs that treat depression, MAO inhibitors, sedatives, or drugs used for psychiatric problems.

- **Drugs that have an anticholinergic effect**

Antihistamines and anticholinergic drugs have similar actions and the combination might be too much. (Anticholinergic drugs are discussed in Chapter 11, page 209)

- **Other antihistamine drugs (because of the added effect)**
- **Aminosalicylic acid**

This drug is sometimes used to treat tuberculosis, and antihistamines may decrease how much of the drug gets absorbed from the stomach.

- **Alcohol**
- **Drugs to control seizures (like phenytoin or Dilantin)**

Some antihistamines may interfere with how the body breaks down these drugs. This means that a very high unsafe blood-level of the anti-seizure medication could develop.

Most of the above drugs (except for alcohol and other antihistamines) are prescription drugs. Therefore, if you are taking any medicine (whether it is prescription or not), before using an over-the-counter drug, talk to your healthcare provider to be sure there is no conflict.

Two Sides of Side Effects

Minor Side Effects

Some minor side effects that you may experience when taking an over-the-counter antihistamine include:

- drowsiness
- tiredness
- clumsiness
- nervousness
- dry mouth or throat
- upset stomach
- nausea
- thicker mucus in the nose or chest areas

If you have questions about these side effects or notice any other unusual feelings, you should talk to your healthcare provider before taking any more of the medicine. Because nausea or an upset stomach can occur with these medications, it is permissible to take them with food. Taking them with food does not seem to affect their antihistamine function but might slow down how quickly they work.

Major Side Effects

If any of the following symptoms develop, you should stop taking the medication immediately and call your healthcare provider right away.

- hallucinations (seeing things or hearing things that other people do not see or hear)
- slurred speech
- severe dizziness or fainting (passing out)
- tremors (shaky hands)
- tachycardia (a very fast heartbeat or heart rate)
- trouble breathing or shortness of breath
- disorientation (not knowing where you are)
- severe sleepiness (difficulty waking up)
- inability to urinate (difficulty emptying the bladder)
- very dilated pupils (the black center part of the eye becomes large and does not shrink very much if exposed to light)

As you can see, many of the major side effects involve the function of the brain or nervous system.

Other Important Facts

Most adults who take these drugs will become tired. However, a few adults and many children will actually do the opposite and become excited or restless.

Since all antihistamines come in a pill or capsule form **you should not crush** them because a greater amount of the drug may be absorbed too quickly from the stomach into the bloodstream which could cause problems.

If you use an antihistamine drug for more than three to four weeks at a time, your body might become resistant to the drug which means that the medication may not be as effective. Therefore, it is recommended that you only use these drugs for no longer than two to three weeks unless you talk with your doctor first.

Allergy Testing

Because antihistamine drugs can be used to fight allergies, if you are going to have allergy tests performed by your healthcare provider, you should not use these drugs before the testing or at least stop using them for a few days prior to testing. The antihistamines may interfere with the test results or give incorrect results.

The Bottom Line

The current list of available antihistamine active ingredients found in over-the-counter medications is as follows:

1. Diphenhydramine
2. Doxylamine
3. Clemastine
4. Chlorpheniramine
5. Dexchlorpheniramine
6. Brompheniramine
7. Dexbrompheniramine
8. Pheniramine
9. Triprolidine
10. Pyrilamine
11. Chlorcyclizine
12. Phenindamine
13. Thonzylamine

If my wife were pregnant and she and I and our doctor decided to use an antihistamine during the pregnancy, I would choose Nos.1, 4 or 2 above (diphenhydramine, chlorpheniramine, or doxylamine) followed very closely by Nos. 9, 5, and 3 (triprolidine, dexchlorpheniramine, or clemastine) because they have been studied the most. This list of 13 drugs (I hope you are not superstitious) was placed in the above sequence because of similarities between some of the antihistamines. Nos. 1, 2, and 3 are similar, Nos. 4 through 9 are similar, Nos. 10, 11 and 12 are in separate categories, and No. 13 is - well, I don't know for sure! Since this book may be used as a reference guide, some information given about each individual drug may be repeated because most of the antihistamines have similar actions.

The Crux of the Matter

This section may seem somewhat technical, but if you have one of the diseases or medical problems listed in the WARNINGS section, this part of the chapter will help to explain why they are listed as warnings. The word antihistamine was briefly introduced in the second paragraph of this chapter as a drug that is anti something called histamine.

Stepping Back Into History

Around 1910, researchers found that if parts of the human body were exposed to a substance (something very common in plants and foods), different reactions in the body would occur. They knew that this substance was a type of chemical called an **amine** (am-MEEN). In 1927, other researchers found that parts of the human body also had this same amine, and shortly thereafter it was given the name **histamine** (histos in Greek means tissue, thus tissue-amine).

For about 40 years (from 1910 to 1950) many studies were performed on histamine and the human body. Researchers learned that histamine would cause the smooth muscle in the lungs to constrict making breathing more difficult and would cause the smooth muscle in the intestines to contract. However, histamine would usually cause the smooth muscle in blood vessels to relax which might decrease or lower blood pressure. Histamine could also cause the stomach to produce more acid and it was also found to bother nerve endings which could cause itching. Finally, researchers learned that histamine could cause tissue and blood vessels to be **more leaky** which would result in swelling and irritation. For easy reference, see Table 5 on page 264 for the effects of histamine on various parts of the body.

For humans, they learned that certain parts of our body (like the lungs, nose, and skin) produce histamine and that some cells inside our body actually store up histamine. If these cells are damaged or are exposed to something that is irritating (like pollen), histamine can be released.

To Pull This All Together

Let's say you are exposed to some irritating pollen in the air which causes your body to release histamine. This histamine release may make it more difficult for you to breathe and may cause an itchy runny nose with itchy watery eyes (hence an allergy-type reaction). The antihistamine drugs try to block some of this effect caused by the released histamine.

Something important for you to know is that anti-histamines DO NOT block the release of histamine. Their purpose is to minimize or lower the effect of the histamine that is about to be released or has already been released.

To explain this further, let's use an example like a nerve ending. If histamine gets to the nerve ending first, itching will occur. However, if the antihistamine gets there first, no itching occurs because the place where the histamine was going to attach on the nerve ending is now filled with the antihistamine, so the histamine reaction does not occur. (Isn't this stuff great?)

Furthermore, your cold or flu is not really an allergy but is a viral infection. It just so happens, as many of you know, that the symptoms of a cold or flu are sometimes similar to the symptoms of an allergy.

In some people, cold or flu viruses may actually cause an allergy-type reaction. In addition, these viruses will cause some cells to die, resulting in the release of histamine and other irritating substances. Therefore, the antihistamines may be helpful in treating your cold or flu symptoms if the symptoms you have are similar to what is described in the first paragraph of this chapter.

A Place To Stay: Receptors

In the 1960s and the 1970s, researchers discovered two different places or **receptors** where histamine can work. These were called H-1 and H-2 receptors (figures, doesn't it?).

However, antihistamines as a class of drugs were originally discovered in the 1940s with two of the first being pyrilamine and diphenhydramine. These two drugs along with the remaining antihistamines in this chapter are all basically H-1 blockers.

Why The Warnings Are Warnings

For those of you with heart disease or high blood pressure, antihistamines do not affect the heart directly. However, they can sometimes change your blood pressure which in turn may affect your heart rate. Therefore, if you have either of these medical conditions, you should talk with your doctor first. Likewise, because blood pressure and heart rate can be affected, people with overactive thyroid glands should also be wary.

If you have diabetes, these drugs do not change blood sugar like the decongestants. However, because they have an effect throughout the body, and because diabetes can affect the body in many places, again you should talk to your healthcare provider first.

People with asthma or chronic bronchitis should consult their doctor prior to using antihistamines. These drugs can make mucus or phlegm (flem) thicker, which could make it more difficult to cough up or remove this material from the lungs.

Because these drugs also have something called an **anticholinergic effect**, people with difficulty urinating or people with narrow-angle glaucoma (an eye problem) should not use these medications without talking to their healthcare provider first.

The reason that liver and kidney problems are listed as warnings is because they are the two main organs in the body which break down and get rid of drugs after they are absorbed. Therefore, if either of these two organs are not functioning properly, the amount of drug or the frequency in which it is used may need adjustment.

The H-1 antihistamines, as a whole, do not seem to affect the blood vessels going to the uterus nor do they act upon the muscles of the uterus itself. Therefore, the effect of these drugs on pregnancy is primarily found in other parts of your body or with the baby.

Finally, the H-1 antihistamines do not block the amount of stomach acid produced by the body. In a few studies involving the H-1 antihistamines, the amount of stomach acid actually increased a little. Because of this, people with stomach or intestinal ulcers should talk to their doctor first.

What About H-2?

In simplified terms, the primary area for H-2 receptors involves the release of stomach acid and some drugs are specifically made to be H-2 blockers which decrease the release of stomach acid. (Just for the record, a new receptor called H-3 has been discovered, but currently no H-3 blocking drugs are available over-the-counter.)

Before using this medication, please read the following :
WARNINGS Section - page 140
DRUG INTERACTIONS Section - page 141
TWO SIDES OF SIDE EFFECTS Section - page 142

1. Diphenhydramine

Diphenhydramine (di-fen-HI-dra-meen) is an anti-histamine found in many over-the-counter cold remedies. If you read a label from an over-the-counter medication that has the word diphenhydramine (only), diphenhydramine hydrochloride, diphenhydramine HCl, or diphenhydramine citrate, they all essentially mean the same. A common brand name (trade name) medication that contains this active ingredient is

Benadryl; however, numerous OTC products contain diphenhydramine. Please remember that the active ingredients in a brand name product can change over time. Therefore, you still need to read the labels.

Of all the antihistamines, diphenhydramine has the largest list of potential uses. It was one of the original antihistamines studied in the 1940s and has been around for over 50 years. Possible uses for this drug other than treating the symptoms of a cold or flu are treating motion sickness, allergic skin reactions, allergic reactions to other foods or drugs, treating insomnia, and treating side effects that occur with some drugs used in psychiatry.

If You Are Pregnant

Diphenhydramine has not been proven to cause major birth defects in humans. From three large studies[1-3], a total of 4,124 pregnant women were identified who took the drug in the first trimester, and no increase in major birth defects was seen over what was expected. In two of these studies[1,2], there were a total of 6,859 women who used this drug at some time in their pregnancy (all three trimesters), and no increase in major birth defects was found. (For statistical information on the number of pregnant women who took this drug in the first trimester compared to other antihistamines, see Table 2 on page 261.)

One study looked at a group of pregnant women who delivered children with a cleft palate defect (the roof of the mouth not completely formed). The number of women who used this drug was higher when compared to pregnancies that did not deliver children with cleft palate. However, this probably represents a population of women with an underlying genetic risk for this birth defect and not a random pregnant population. This birth defect was not found to be increased in the other large general pregnant population studies.

There is also one report of a baby that died before birth (stillbirth). The mother took this drug along with a prescription tranquilizer. No one can know for sure whether combining this drug with the tranquilizer caused the stillbirth. However, the message here is that **you should not mix** antihistamines with tranquilizers or other drugs that are sedating (especially while pregnant).

Another important message about this drug is that nearly four million women give birth each year in the United States, and some of these women will have an allergic reaction to a food, drug, or bug bite. Diphenhydramine is often used to counteract that allergic reaction. Therefore, this drug is commonly used by pregnant women and no major problems have been reported in the general pregnant population.

Finally, this drug has been studied in pregnant animals that were given doses larger than those recommended for humans and no harm was identified.

Some medical specialists have classified diphenhydramine as a pregnancy risk category B while others have listed it as a C. I would categorize this drug as a B for its use as an over-the-counter medication (see Chapter 4, How is Drug Safety Determined?).

No long-term effects that may show up later in life have been reported with the use of this drug during pregnancy.

Details About Diphenhydramine

- For dosing information, read the package material carefully because all drugs vary on the amount that can be used and the frequency of their use.
- The onset of action (when you might see some response) is usually within about one hour of taking the medicine.
- The duration of action (how long the effect might last) is about four to six hours.
- The absorption (how much is taken into the bloodstream) occurs in the intestines and the majority of the oral dose is absorbed.
- The metabolism of the drug (how the body breaks down the drug) occurs in the liver and the majority of the drug is eventually broken down.
- The elimination of the drug (how the body gets rid of it) is accomplished by the kidneys.
- The half-life of the drug (the amount of time it takes the body to remove half of the drug still circulating in the bloodstream) is about four to eight hours.

Other Information

This drug is also marketed in some nasal sprays and, therefore, the same precautions with nasal sprays should be followed (see pages 96-98).

Diphenhydramine and doxylamine (No. 2) are probably the most sedating antihistamines available over-the-counter. In fact, most of the OTC drugs used in combating **insomnia** contain diphenhydramine. Therefore, this probably is the major drawback to using this antihistamine, especially if taken during the daytime.

This drug also comes in a cream form which can be used for treating allergic skin reactions. It is very important that this cream be used with caution on open sores, cuts, or blisters because the drug can be absorbed into the bloodstream through these locations and high blood levels have been reported. This problem has primarily been seen in people who rubbed the cream over a large area of sores or blisters (like chicken pox). Therefore, if you use this cream, be sure to only apply it to a limited area or talk to your doctor first.

Breast-feeding

No thorough studies on breast-feeding and this drug have been reported. The drug can be found in breast milk, but the amount is probably low and the effect on a baby is not fully known. The manufacturers, however, do not recommend the use of this drug while breast-feeding because of possible problems for the newborn such as sedation, sleepiness, or fussiness.

Before using this medication, please read the following :
WARNINGS Section - page 140
DRUG INTERACTIONS Section - page 141
TWO SIDES OF SIDE EFFECTS Section - page 142

2. Doxylamine

Doxylamine (dox-ILL-am-meen) is another antihistamine found in over-the-counter cold remedies. If you read a label from an over-the-counter medication that has the word doxylamine (only) or doxylamine succinate, they essentially mean the same. A common brand name (trade name) medication that contains this active ingredient is Vicks Nyquil. However, please remember that the active ingredients in a brand name product can change over time. Therefore, you still need to read the labels.

Because this antihistamine is in the same category as diphenhydramine, one of the major side effects is sedation. This drug, however, lasts longer than diphenhydramine and a few people have described a hangover effect (not like an alcohol hangover) meaning it occasionally lasts into the next day.

If You Are Pregnant

Unfortunately, nausea and vomiting are a common problem in pregnancy. Over the years, many different ways of treating this problem have been tried. Over 15 years ago, one method of treating nausea in pregnancy was with a drug called Bendectin which originally contained doxylamine, dicyclomine (DI-sigh-clo-meen, an anticholinergic-type drug) and pyridoxine (peer-uh-DOX-een) which is vitamin B6. Bendectin was first marketed in 1956, but in 1976 the components of the drug were changed by the manufacturer. The dicyclomine portion was removed because it was not considered necessary in treating nausea. Over 33 million women used this drug in pregnancy to treat their nausea and the preponderance of these exposures were during the first trimester when most of the nausea of pregnancy occurs. The vast majority of these reports showed no increase in major birth defects over what was expected.

The company that produced Bendectin eventually took it off the market in 1983 because it was spending more money defending the drug in court than in profiting from sales.

Doxylamine has probably been the most extensively studied drug in human pregnancy. From three large studies[1-3] alone, a total of 10,998 first trimester exposures were identified, and no increase in major birth defects was seen over what was expected. After analyzing multiple reports, the U.S. Food and Drug Administration **concluded that this drug was probably not a teratogen**. The manufacturer considers its use contraindicated in pregnancy, whereas most other medical specialists (including myself) have classified doxylamine as a pregnancy risk category B (see Chapter 4, How is Drug Safety Determined?).

No long-term effects that may show up later in life have been reported with the use of this drug during pregnancy.

Doxylamine is approved for over-the-counter use in treating cold or flu symptoms and as a nighttime sleep-aid. According to the manufacturer, this drug is not approved for the treatment of nausea in pregnancy. Because doxylamine is one of the most sedating antihistamines, it is not a preferred choice by many people for daytime use.

Details About Doxylamine

- For dosing information, read the package material carefully because all drugs vary on the amount that can be used and the frequency of their use.
- The onset of action (when you might see some response) is usually within about 30 minutes of taking the medicine.
- The duration of action (how long the effect might last) is about five to ten hours.
- The absorption (how much is taken into the bloodstream) occurs in the intestines and most of an oral dose is absorbed.
- The metabolism of the drug (how the body breaks down the drug) occurs in the liver and the majority of the drug is eventually broken down.

- The elimination of the drug (how the body gets rid of it) is accomplished by the kidneys.
- The half-life of the drug (the amount of time it takes the body to remove half of the drug still circulating in the bloodstream) is about ten to twelve hours.

Breast-feeding

No thorough studies on breast-feeding and this drug have been reported. Doxylamine can probably be found in breast milk. However, the amount of drug and what effect it may have on the baby is unknown.

Before using this medication, please read the following :
WARNINGS Section - page 140
DRUG INTERACTIONS Section - page 141
TWO SIDES OF SIDE EFFECTS Section - page 142

3. Clemastine

Clemastine (clee-MAST-teen) is another antihistamine found in over-the-counter cold remedies. If you read a label from an over-the-counter medication that has the word clemastine (only) or clemastine fumarate, they essentially mean the same. A common brand name (trade name) medication that contains this active ingredient is Tavist. However, please remember that the active ingredients in a brand name product can change over time. Therefore, you still need to read the labels.

This drug is similar to Nos. 1 and 2 (diphenhydramine and doxylamine) but is reported to be less sedating. Therefore, it is not used to treat insomnia. However, all antihistamines can make people sleepy and, therefore, the same precautions should be taken. Clemastine was originally a prescription drug but was switched to over-the-counter use in 1992. This antihistamine is also considered long-acting and is usually only taken twice a day.

If You Are Pregnant

Clemastine has not been proven to cause major birth defects in humans. One study[2] identified 1,831 pregnant women who used clemastine in the first trimester, and no increase in major birth defects was seen over what was expected. (For statistical information on the number of pregnant women who took this drug in the first trimester compared to other antihistamines, see Table 2 on page 261.) This drug has also been studied in pregnant animals that were given doses much larger than those recommended for humans and no harmful effects were identified.

The manufacturer has listed this drug as category B. However, I would classify clemastine as have other medical specialists, as a pregnancy risk category C (see Chapter 4, How is Drug Safety Determined?).

No long-term effects that may show up later in life have been reported with the use of this drug during pregnancy.

Details About Clemastine

- For dosing information, read the package material carefully because all drugs vary on the amount that can be used and the frequency of their use.

- The onset of action (when you might see some response) is usually within about two hours of taking the medicine.

- The duration of action (how long the effect might last) is about ten to twelve hours, but may last up to 24 hours in some people.
- The absorption (how much is taken into the bloodstream) occurs in the intestines and most of an oral dose is absorbed according to the manufacturer.
- The metabolism of the drug (how the body breaks down the drug) occurs in the liver and the majority of the drug is eventually broken down.
- The elimination of the drug (how the body gets rid of it) is accomplished by the kidneys.
- The half-life of the drug (the amount of time it takes the body to remove half of the drug still circulating in the bloodstream) is about 21 hours.

Breast-feeding

Very few reports on breast-feeding with this drug can be found. There is one report of a baby that became sleepy and irritable after the mother started this drug, but she was also using other medicines that could cause sleepiness. The American Academy of Pediatrics states that this drug should be used with caution while breast-feeding.

Before using this medication, please read the following :
WARNINGS Section - page 140
DRUG INTERACTIONS Section - page 141
TWO SIDES OF SIDE EFFECTS Section - page 142

4. Chlorpheniramine & 5. Dexchlorpheniramine

Chlorpheniramine (KLOR-fen-ear-am-meen) and dexchlorpheniramine (DEX-klor-fen-ear-am-meen) are both antihistamines that can be found in over-the-counter cold remedies. If you read a label that has the word chlorpheniramine (only) or chlorpheniramine maleate, they essentially mean the same. Likewise, the word dexchlorpheniramine (only) or dexchlorpheniramine maleate also essentially mean the same.

A common brand name (trade name) for chlorpheniramine is Chlor-Trimeton; however, numerous OTC products contain this active ingredient. Please remember that the active ingredients in a brand name product can change over time. Therefore, you still need to read the labels.

You may wonder why I listed these two drugs together. As I have said before, all of the antihistamines are similar, but these two are very similar. Chlorpheniramine and dexchlorpheniramine are **mirror image** drugs. The subject of mirror image drugs was discused in detail under Levmetamfetamine, pages 133-134. For the sake of clarity, if we put chlorpheniramine in front of a mirror, the drug staring back from the mirror would be dexchlorpheniramine. Chlorpheniramine is really levo-chlorpheniramine and dexchlorpheniramine is really dextro-chlorpheniramine. However, in order to make things easier, the levo part is dropped leaving you with chlorpheniramine and dextrochlorpheniramine is shortened a little to dexchlorpheniramine. Remember, mirror image drugs do not always work the same.

To repeat a prior example, let's say there is a pain medicine called "levo-pain" so its mirror image is "dextro-pain." "Levo-pain" may work very well in taking away your pain. However, "dextro-pain" could be stronger, could be the same, could be weaker, or might have no action whatsoever when compared to "levo-pain."

For chlorpheniramine and dexchlorpheniramine, when comparing equal amounts of drug, dexchlorpheniramine is about twice as strong as chlorpheniramine. These two antihistamines are similar to Nos. 6, 7, 8, and 9 in this chapter and are supposed to be less sedating than Nos. 1 and 2 (diphenhydramine and doxylamine). However, these drugs can still be very sedating for some people and, therefore, the same precautions should be taken.

If You Are Pregnant

Neither chlorpheniramine nor dexchlorpheniramine have been proven to cause major birth defects in humans. For **chlorpheniramine**, three large studies[1-3] identified at least 2,581 pregnant women who used the drug in the first trimester, and no increase in major birth defects was seen over what was expected. In two of these studies[1,2], a total of 4,168 women used chlorpheniramine at some time in their pregnancy (all three trimesters), and no increase in major birth defects was identified. (For statistical information on the number of pregnant women who took this drug in the first trimester compared to other antihistamines, see Table 2 on page 261.)

This drug has been studied in pregnant animals that were given doses larger than those recommended for humans and no harm was identified.

For **dexchlorpheniramine**, one study[2] identified 1,080 pregnant women who used this drug in the first trimester, and no increase in major birth defects was seen over what was expected. In this same study, a total of 2,275 pregnant women used the drug at some time in their pregnancy (all three trimesters), and no increase in major birth defects was found.

Most manufacturers have classified both of these as a pregnancy risk category B. More information exists for chlorpheniramine, and I would agree with the category B classification based on the current data. Because dexchlorpheniramine is so similar to chlorpheniramine (except that it is stronger) it also has been labeled as a B (see Chapter 4, How is Drug Safety Determined?).

No long-term effects that may show up later in life have been reported with the use of these drugs during pregnancy.

Details About Chlorpheniramine and Dexchlorpheniramine

- For dosing information, read the package material carefully because all drugs vary on the amount that can be used and the frequency of their use.

- The onset of action (when you might see some response) is usually within about 30 minutes for both drugs.

- The duration of action (how long the effect might last) is about three to six hours for both drugs.
- The absorption (how much is taken into the bloodstream) occurs in the intestines and most of an oral dose is absorbed for both drugs.
- The metabolism of each drug (how the body breaks down the drug) occurs in the liver and the majority of both drugs is eventually broken down.
- The elimination of each drug (how the body gets rid of it) is accomplished by the kidneys.
- The half-life of each drug (the amount of time it takes the body to remove half of the drug still circulating in the bloodstream) is about 20 hours.

Other Information

Both of these drugs have the same action. However, when you read the label for how much drug is found in a pill, you will often see that the amount for dexchlorpheniramine is about half of that for chlorpheniramine. This is because dexchlorpheniramine is twice as strong.

Breast-feeding

No thorough studies on breast-feeding and these drugs have been reported. Both of these can probably be found in breast milk, but the amount of drug and what effect it may have on the baby is unknown.

Before using this medication, please read the following :
WARNINGS Section - page 140
DRUG INTERACTIONS Section - page 141
TWO SIDES OF SIDE EFFECTS Section - page 142

6. Brompheniramine & 7. Dexbrompheniramine

Brompheniramine (BROM-fen-ear-am-meen) and dexbrompheniramine (DEX-brom-fen-ear-am-meen) are both antihistamines that can be found in over-the-counter cold remedies. If you read a label that has the word brompheniramine (only) or brompheniramine maleate, they essentially mean the same. Likewise, the word dexbrompheniramine (only) or dexbrompheniramine maleate also essentially mean the same.

A common brand name (trade name) product that contains brompheniramine is Dimetapp. A common brand name medication that contains dexbrompheniramine is Drixoral. However, please remember that the active ingredients in a brand name product can change over time. Therefore, you still need to read the labels.

These two antihistamines are **mirror images** (fully discussed in the section about Levmetamfetamine, pages 133-134.) Therefore, this mirror image thing is the same for these two drugs. In addition, when comparing equal amounts of drug, dexbrompheniramine is a little stronger than brompheniramine. These two antihistamines are similar to Nos. 4, 5, 8, and 9 in this chapter and are supposed to be less sedating than Nos. 1 and 2 (diphenhydramine and doxylamine). However, these drugs can still be very sedating for some people and, therefore, the same precautions should be taken.

If You Are Pregnant

Neither brompheniramine nor dexbrompheniramine have truly been proven to cause major birth defects in humans. For **brompheniramine**, one study[1] identified 65 pregnant women who used the drug in the first trimester, and an **increase** in overall birth defects was seen over what was expected, but there was **no pattern** to the defects. In the same study, there were 412 women who used this drug at some time in their pregnancy (all three trimesters), and no increase in major birth defects was seen over what was expected. In two other large studies[2,3], a total of at least 1,131 first trimester exposures were recorded, and no increase in major birth defects was found. (For statistical information on the number of pregnant women who took this drug in the first trimester compared to other antihistamines, see Table 2 on page 261.) This drug has been studied in pregnant animals that were given doses larger than those recommended for humans and no harm was identified.

For **dexbrompheniramine**, one large study[2] identified a total of 471 pregnant women with first trimester exposure, and no increase in major birth defects was identified. Another study[1] identified 14 first trimester exposures, but exact details regarding outcome were not supplied.

These drugs have been classified by some medical specialists as a pregnancy risk category B while others have classified them as a C (see Chapter 4, How is Drug Safety Determined?). I would list these drugs as category C because not as much information is available compared to the other antihistamines.

No long-term effects that may show up later in life have been reported with the use of these drugs during pregnancy.

Details About Brompheniramine and Dexbrompheniramine

- For dosing information, read the package material carefully because all drugs vary on the amount that can be used and the frequency of their use.
- The onset of action (when you might see some response) is usually within about 30 minutes to an hour for both drugs.
- The duration of action (how long the effect might last) is about four to six hours for both drugs.
- The absorption (how much is taken into the bloodstream) occurs in the intestines and most of an oral dose is absorbed for both drugs.
- The metabolism of each drug (how the body breaks down the drug) occurs in the liver and the majority of both drugs is eventually broken down.
- The elimination of each drug (how the body gets rid of it) is accomplished by the kidneys.
- The half-life of each drug (the amount of time it takes the body to remove half of the drug still circulating in the bloodstream) is about 25 hours.

Other Information

Both of these drugs have the same action. However, when you read the label for how much drug is found in a sustained-release pill, you may see that the amount for dexbrompheniramine is less than that for brompheniramine. This is because dexbrompheniramine is a little stronger.

Breast-feeding

No thorough studies on breast-feeding and these drugs have been reported. There is one report of a baby that became irritable with a lot of crying and sleeping problems when the mother was using a cold medicine that had brompheniramine with a decongestant. When the mother stopped the drug, the symptoms in the baby improved. Some people have said that brompheniramine should not be used while breast-feeding. However, the American Academy of Pediatrics states that breast-feeding while taking dexbrompheniramine is acceptable. In all honesty, there is very little information about these drugs and breast-feeding. If a problem were to occur while using these drugs at the recommended dosage and frequency, more than likely it would be similar to the baby described above.

Before using this medication, please read the following :
WARNINGS Section - page 140
DRUG INTERACTIONS Section - page 141
TWO SIDES OF SIDE EFFECTS Section - page 142

8. Pheniramine

Pheniramine (FEN-ear-am-meen) is another antihistamine found in over-the-counter cold remedies. If you read a label from one of the OTC medications and you see the word pheniramine (only) or pheniramine maleate, they essentially mean the same.

Pheniramine is similar to Nos. 4, 5, 6, 7, and 9 in this chapter and is supposed to be less sedating than Nos. 1 and 2 (diphenhydramine and doxylamine). However, this drug can still be very sedating for some people and, therefore, the same precautions should be taken.

If You Are Pregnant

Pheniramine has not been proven to cause major birth defects in humans. One study[1] identified 831 pregnant women who used this drug in the first trimester, and no increase in major birth defects was seen over what was expected. In the same study, a total of 2,442 women used this medication at some time in their pregnancy (all three trimesters), and no increase in major birth defects was identified. (For statistical information on the number of pregnant women who took this drug in the first trimester compared to other antihistamines, see Table 2 on page 261.) Animal studies during pregnancy on this particular drug were not found.

Despite the above information, this drug would still be classified according to the pregnancy risk category as a C (see Chapter 4, How is Drug Safety Determined?).

No long-term effects that may show up later in life have been reported with the use of this drug during pregnancy.

Details About Pheniramine

- For dosing information, read the package material carefully because all drugs vary on the amount that can be used and the frequency of their use.
- The onset of action (when you might see some response) is usually within about one to two hours.
- The duration of action (how long the effect might last) is about four to six hours.
- The absorption (how much is taken into the bloodstream) occurs in the intestines and most of an oral dose is absorbed.

- The metabolism of the drug (how the body breaks down the drug) occurs in the liver and the majority of the drug is eventually broken down.
- The elimination of the drug (how the body gets rid of it) is accomplished by the kidneys.
- The half-life of the drug (the amount of time it takes the body to remove half of the drug still circulating in the bloodstream) is about 16 to 19 hours.

Other Information

This drug is also marketed in some nasal sprays and, therefore, the same precautions with nasal sprays should be followed (see pages 96-98).

Breast-feeding

No thorough studies on breast-feeding and this drug have been reported. Pheniramine can probably be found in breast milk. However, the amount of drug and what effect it may have on the baby is unknown.

Before using this medication, please read the following :
WARNINGS Section - page 140
DRUG INTERACTIONS Section - page 141
TWO SIDES OF SIDE EFFECTS Section - page 142

9. Triprolidine

Triprolidine (tri-PRO-leh-deen) is another antihistamine found in over-the-counter cold remedies. If you read a label from one of the OTC medications and you see the word triprolidine (only), triprolidine hydrochloride, or triprolidine HCl, they essentially mean the same. A common brand name (trade name) medication that contains this active ingredient is Actifed. However, please remember that the active ingredients in a brand name product can change over time. Therefore, you still need to read the labels.

Triprolidine is similar to Nos. 4, 5, 6, 7, and 8 in this chapter and is supposed to be less sedating than Nos. 1 and 2 (diphenhydramine and doxylamine). However, this drug can still be very sedating for some people and, therefore, the same precautions should be taken.

If You Are Pregnant

Triprolidine has not been proven to cause major birth defects in humans. From two large studies[2,3], a total of 1,538 pregnant women were identified who took this drug in the first trimester, and no increase in major birth defects was seen over what was expected. A third study[1] identified 16 pregnancies with first trimester exposure but exact details regarding outcome were not supplied. (For statistical information on the number of pregnant women who took this drug in the first trimester compared to other antihistamines, see Table 2 on page 261.) According to the manufacturer, this drug has been studied in pregnant animals that were given doses larger than those recommended for humans and no harm was identified.

Despite the above information, this drug would still be classified according to the pregnancy risk category as a C (see Chapter 4, How is Drug Safety Determined?).

No long-term effects that may show up later in life have been reported with the use of this drug during pregnancy.

Details About Triprolidine

- For dosing information, read the package material carefully because all drugs vary on the amount that can be used and the frequency of their use.
- The onset of action (when you might see some response) is usually about 30 minutes after taking the medicine.
- The duration of action (how long the effect might last) is about two to six hours.
- The absorption (how much is taken into the bloodstream) occurs in the intestines and most of an oral dose is absorbed according to the manufacturer.
- The metabolism of the drug (how the body breaks down the drug) occurs in the liver and the majority of the drug is eventually broken down.
- The elimination of the drug (how the body gets rid of it) is accomplished by the kidneys.
- The half-life of the drug (the amount of time it takes the body to remove half of the drug still circulating in the bloodstream) is about two to five hours.

Breast-feeding

No thorough studies on breast-feeding and this drug have been reported. Triprolidine can be found in the milk. However, the amount of drug in the few samples studied to date was very small and would probably have little or no effect on a baby. The American Academy of Pediatrics states that breast-feeding while using triprolidine is acceptable.

Before using this medication, please read the following :
WARNINGS Section - page 140
DRUG INTERACTIONS Section - page 141
TWO SIDES OF SIDE EFFECTS Section - page 142

10. Pyrilamine

Pyrilamine (per-ILL-am-meen) is another antihistamine found in over-the-counter cold remedies. If you read a label from one of the OTC medications and you see the word pyrilamine (only) or pyrilamine maleate, they essentially mean the same.

This active ingredient is in a group by itself and is a little different from the other antihistamines in this chapter. This drug can still be very sedating for some people and, therefore, the same precautions should be taken.

If You Are Pregnant

Pyrilamine has not been proven to cause major birth defects in humans. One study[1] identified 121 pregnant women who used this drug in the first trimester, and no increase in major birth defects was seen over what was expected. In the same study, there were 392 women who used this medication at some time in their pregnancy (all three trimesters), and no increase in major birth defects was identified. (For statistical information on the number of pregnant women who took this drug in the first trimester compared to other antihistamines, see Table 2 on page 261.) Animal studies during pregnancy on this particular drug were not found.

This drug would be classified according to the pregnancy risk category as a C (see Chapter 4, How is Drug Safety Determined?).

No long-term effects that may show up later in life have been reported with the use of this drug during pregnancy.

Details About Pyrilamine

No significant details on this drug could be obtained regarding onset of action, duration of action, and half-life. The drug is metabolized by the liver, and the kidneys eliminate it from the body whether it is metabolized or not. Very few over-the-counter cold remedies contain pyrilamine.

This drug is also marketed in some nasal sprays and, therefore, the same precautions with nasal sprays should be followed (see pages 96-98).

Breast-feeding

No thorough studies on breast-feeding and this drug have been reported. Pyrilamine can probably be found in breast milk. However, the amount of drug and what effect it may have on the baby is unknown.

Before using this medication, please read the following :
WARNINGS Section - page 140
DRUG INTERACTIONS Section - page 141
TWO SIDES OF SIDE EFFECTS Section - page 142

11. Chlorcyclizine

Chlorcyclizine (klor-SYE-cleh-zeen) is another antihistamine found in over-the-counter cold remedies. If you read a label from one of the OTC medications and you see the word chlorcyclizine (only), chlorcyclizine hydrochloride, or chlorcyclizine HCl, they essentially mean the same.

This antihistamine is also in a group by itself and is a little different from the other antihistamines in this chapter. This drug can still be very sedating for some people and, therefore, the same precautions should be taken.

If You Are Pregnant

Chlorcyclizine has not been proven to cause major birth defects in humans. Only 13 pregnant women were identified in one study[1] who took this drug in the first trimester, and exact details regarding outcome were not supplied. (For statistical information on the number of pregnant women who took this drug in the first trimester compared to other antihistamines, see Table 2 on page 261.) Animal studies during pregnancy on this particular drug were not found.

This drug would be classified according to the pregnancy risk category as a C (see Chapter 4, How is Drug Safety Determined?).

No long-term effects that may show up later in life have been reported with the use of this drug during pregnancy.

Details About Chlorcyclizine

No significant details on this drug could be obtained regarding onset of action, duration of action, and half-life. The drug is metabolized by the liver, and the kidneys eliminate it from the body whether it is metabolized or not. Very few over-the-counter cold remedies contain chlorcyclizine.

Breast-feeding

No thorough studies on breast-feeding and this drug have been reported. Chlorcyclizine can probably be found in breast milk. However, the amount of drug and what effect it may have on the baby is unknown.

Before using this medication, please read the following :
WARNINGS Section - page 140
DRUG INTERACTIONS Section - page 141
TWO SIDES OF SIDE EFFECTS Section - page 142

12. Phenindamine

Phenindamine (FEN-in-duh-meen) is another antihistamine found in over-the-counter cold remedies. If you read a label from one of the OTC medications and you see the word phenindamine (only) or phenindamine tartrate, they essentially mean the same.

According to the manufacturer, this antihistamine does not fit into any category exclusively and is therefore labeled miscellaneous. This drug can still be very sedating for some people and, therefore, the same precautions should be taken.

If You Are Pregnant

Phenindamine has not been proven to cause major birth defects in humans. Only 12 pregnant women were identified in one study[1] who took this drug in the first trimester, and exact details regarding outcome were not supplied. (For statistical information on the number of pregnant women who took this drug in the first trimester compared to other antihistamines, see Table 2 on page 261.) Animal studies during pregnancy on this particular drug were not found.

This drug would be classified according to the pregnancy risk category as a C (see Chapter 4, How is Drug Safety Determined?).

No long-term effects that may show up later in life have been reported with the use of this drug during pregnancy.

Details About Phenindamine

No significant details on this drug could be obtained regarding onset of action, duration of action, and half-life. The drug is metabolized by the liver, and the kidneys eliminate it from the body whether it is metabolized or not. Very few over-the-counter cold remedies contain phenindamine.

Breast-feeding

No thorough studies on breast-feeding and this drug have been reported. Phenindamine can probably be found in breast milk. However, the amount of drug and what effect it may have on the baby is unknown.

Before using this medication, please read the following :
WARNINGS Section - page 140
DRUG INTERACTIONS Section - page 141
TWO SIDES OF SIDE EFFECTS Section - page 142

13. Thonzylamine

According to the FDA, thonzylamine (thon-ZIL-am-meen) is an antihistamine that may be found in over-the-counter cold remedies. However, I could not find any over-the-counter drugs that contained this active ingredient, and it is possible that this drug is no longer marketed in the United States. In searching several medical libraries, thonzylamine was first mentioned in the Physicians' Desk Reference (PDR) in the early 1950s. It then was listed as a non-prescription medication in the 1970s. The last PDR in which I could find this drug referenced was 1980.

In case this drug is available somewhere in the U.S., if you read a label from an OTC medication and you see the word thonzylamine (only), thonzylamine hydrochloride, or thonzylamine HCl, they essentially mean the same. Because this drug is an antihistamine (all of which have some levels of sedation), the same precautions should be taken.

If You Are Pregnant

Thonzylamine has not been proven to cause major birth defects in humans. One study[1] identified 148 pregnant women who took this drug in the first trimester, and no increase in major birth defects was seen over what was expected. In the same study, there were 444 women who used this drug at some time in their pregnancy (all three trimesters), and no increase in major birth defects was seen. (For statistical information on the number of pregnant women who took this drug in the first trimester compared to other antihistamines, see Table 2 on page 261.) Animal studies during pregnancy on this particular drug were not found.

This drug would be classified according to the pregnancy risk category as a C (see Chapter 4, How is Drug Safety Determined?).

No long-term effects that may show up later in life have been reported with the use of this drug during pregnancy.

Details About Thonzylamine

No significant details on this drug could be obtained regarding onset of action, duration of action, and half-life. The drug is probably metabolized by the liver, and the kidneys probably eliminate it from the body whether it is metabolized or not. As stated above, I could not find any over-the-counter cold remedies containing thonzylamine.

Breast-feeding

No thorough studies on breast-feeding and this drug have been reported. Thonzylamine can probably be found in breast milk. However, the amount of drug and what effect it may have on the baby is unknown.

9. Expectorants

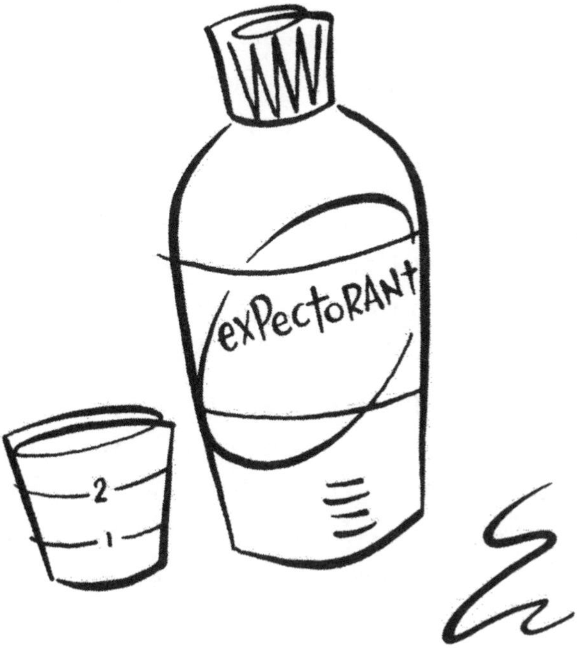

Expectorants are a class of drugs that are supposed to make mucus or phlegm in the lungs thinner so it can be coughed up easier. Some of the FDA recommended ways of describing what these medications may do are: loosen phlegm, thin bronchial secretions, rid the bronchial passageways of bothersome mucus, help drain the bronchial tubes and/or make coughs more productive. These drugs do not work on suppressing the cough itself (see Chapter 10). However, if you are coughing and the material you are bringing up is thick or is hard to get out, expectorants TRY to make this easier.

A Job Made Easier

Before I proceed, I should tell you that the U.S. Food and Drug Administration has made my job in this chapter very easy. The reason I say this is because according to the FDA, only one (yes, only one) drug has been approved as an over-the-counter expectorant. Before the FDA began reviewing drugs in a thorough systematic fashion, there were over 15 different chemicals or drugs that were listed as having expectorant properties. When the FDA finished its review, only one was left. What they discovered was that for most people (excluding pregnant women for now) the 15 or so drugs were not considered to be effective. In other words, they could not be proven to work as expectorants.

The only approved drug for use as an expectorant is guaifenesin which is discussed below. If my wife were pregnant, and she and I and our doctor decided to use an expectorant during the pregnancy, guaifenesin is the one we would choose, and this was true even before the others were removed from an OTC status.

Because there is only one approved expectorant, information regarding warnings, drug interactions, and side effects will be covered under the individual drug.

This chapter also includes small sections on **potassium iodide, iodinated glycerol** and **ammonium chloride** which used to be marketed as expectorants but are no longer approved by the FDA for use over-the-counter. These ingredients could be a problem for pregnant women, and may still be found in **natural products** (marketed as cold remedies).

Finally, when should a person consider using an expectorant? Most experts agree that an expectorant would have the best effect when used with nonproductive coughs (coughs where nothing comes up) or coughs with thick, sticky mucus that only comes up in small amounts. An expectorant is supposed to thin out the mucus and potentially increase the amount that is brought up.

Guaifenesin

Guaifenesin (gwy-FEN-eh-sin) is the only FDA approved over-the-counter expectorant. If you read a label from an over-the-counter medication that has the word guaifenesin or glyceryl guaiacolate (glih-SER-ill) (gwy-AK-o-late), they essentially mean the same thing. A common brand name (trade name) drug that contains this active ingredient is Robitussin. However, please remember that the active ingredients in a brand name product can change over time. Therefore, you still need to read the labels.

This drug does not seem to affect many parts of the body and there are few warnings listed. It might cause an upset stomach in some individuals, and the FDA also states that this drug is not to be used by people such as smokers or those with chronic lung problems such as asthma, chronic bronchitis, or emphysema. Furthermore, there do not appear to be any drug interactions with this active ingredient by itself. Remember, many of the over-the-counter cold remedies are a combination of active ingredients and, therefore, if the medicine you are about to take has guaifenesin combined with something else, you should check for drug interactions of the other active ingredients.

If You Are Pregnant

Guaifenesin has not been proven to cause major birth defects in humans. From three large studies[1-3], a total of at least 1,078 pregnant women were identified who took this drug in the first trimester, and no increase in major birth defects was seen over what was expected. In two of these studies[1,2], there were a total of 1,685 women who used this drug at some time in their pregnancy (all three trimesters), and no increase in major birth defects was found. (For statistical information on the number of pregnant women who took this drug in the first trimester, see Table 3 on page 262.) Animal studies during pregnancy on this particular drug were not found.

Despite the above information, this drug would still be classified according to the pregnancy risk category as a C (see Chapter 4, How is Drug Safety Determined?).

No long-term effects that may show up later in life have been reported with the use of this drug during pregnancy.

Details About Guaifenesin

For dosing information, read the package material carefully because all drugs vary on the amount that can be used and the frequency of their use. No significant details on this drug could be obtained regarding onset of action, duration of action, and half-life. Absorption of this medication occurs in the intestines and most of an oral dose is absorbed. The metabolism of guaifenesin occurs partly in the bloodstream but mostly in the liver. The elimination of the drug is accomplished by the kidneys.

One interesting fact about this medication is there have been a few studies analyzing the use of guaifenesin to thin out the mucus of a woman's cervix in couples who are having infertility problems. One of the listed causes for infertility in some couples is thick mucus of the cervix which may cause difficulties for sperm to pass. However, if you have infertility problems, do not take this medication without talking to your infertility specialist first.

Breast-feeding

No thorough studies on breast-feeding and this drug have been reported. This drug probably can be found in breast milk, but the amount and what effect it may have on the baby is unknown.

Potassium Iodide and Iodinated Glycerol

Potassium iodide and iodinated glycerol are no longer approved by the FDA as over-the-counter expectorants because they are not considered effective. However, as stated in the beginning of this chapter, potassium iodide, iodinated glycerol, and other iodide-containing medications **may be found in natural remedies** used for treating cold symptoms. In addition, some of these ingredients **may still be found in prescription drugs**.

Potassium iodide is used in hospitals to treat people suffering from a severe form of an overactive thyroid gland (often prior to surgery). Therefore, as you might guess, this drug can affect the thyroid gland.

The mineral iodine plays a major role in the makeup of thyroid hormone. Conversely, iodide chemicals can hamper the production of thyroid hormone. It is important to understand, however, that the thyroid gland of an unborn baby does not actually use iodine until after the first trimester (after 12 weeks' gestation).

If you are pregnant, iodide chemicals (including potassium iodide and iodinated glycerol) **can cross over to the baby**. These iodide ingredients are a main concern if used by a mother in the second or third trimester because they can affect the function of the baby's thyroid gland. Because of this effect, these ingredients are **NOT recommended for use in pregnancy**.

If used in the first trimester, iodide medications have not been proven to cause major birth defects. One study[1] identified 56 women with first trimester exposure to potassium iodide and a total of 489 pregnant women who used iodides in general in the first trimester, and no increase in major birth defects was seen over what was expected. In this same study, a total of 221 pregnant women used potassium iodide and 1,635 used iodides in general at some time in their pregnancy (all three trimesters), and no increase in major birth defects was identified.

For iodinated glycerol, one study[2] recorded 1,453 women with first trimester exposure to this drug, and no increase in major birth defects was seen over what was expected. In this same study, 2,617 pregnant women used the medication at some time in their pregnancy (all three trimesters), and no increase in major birth defects was identified.

Because of the potential effect on the baby's thyroid gland, iodinated glycerol would probably be classified according to the pregnancy risk category as an X (see Chapter 4, How is Drug Safety Determined?). This is because it could adversely affect the baby and it has no use in pregnancy. Potassium iodide would be classified as a D because it might be used in rare circumstances in some pregnancies. If a pregnant women has a severe case of an overactive thyroid gland, potassium iodide might be temporarily used as part of the treatment. If the baby were to have a low level of thyroid hormone following delivery, this could be appropriately treated.

Another fact you should know about iodide-containing products is that they may interact with some prescription drugs, and too much iodide may cause irregular heartbeats, confusion, and numbness or tingling in the arms and legs.

The American Academy of Pediatrics has reported that iodide medications can be found in breast milk and could affect a baby's thyroid gland. However, despite this finding, if the recommended dose and frequency of the iodide medication is followed, breast-feeding is considered acceptable.

Ammonium Chloride

Ammonium chloride is no longer approved by the FDA as an over-the-counter expectorant because it is not considered to be effective. However, as stated in the beginning of the chapter, this drug may be found in **natural remedies** used for treating cold symptoms. In addition, this ingredient is still found in prescription medications.

Ammonium chloride is used in hospitals to treat people who have a rare blood/urine problem involving something called pH (discussed below). Ammonium chloride has not been proven to cause major birth defects in humans. One study[1] identified 365 pregnant women who took this drug in the first trimester, and no increase in major birth defects was seen over what was expected. In this same study, there were 3,401 women who used the drug at some time in their pregnancy (all three trimesters), and no increase in major birth defects was identified. Ammonium chloride would be classified according to the pregnancy risk category as a C (see Chapter 4, How is Drug Safety Determined?).

As stated above, this drug can work on something called pH. The human body, if working normally, has a pH of about 7.4. (Remember, pH is a measure that relates the balance between acids and bases. The pH scale ranges from 0 to 14 with battery acid close to 0, neutral close to 7, and lye close to 14.) This means there is a balance between acids and bases in our blood and tissues. If a person's acid/base balance is abnormal, this drug might be used in hospitals to treat the problem. The reason for discussing this topic is because there have been a few reports of pregnant women who took too much of this drug (when it was available over-the-counter) and developed a condition called **acidosis** which adversely affected the health of their babies.

To conclude, ammonium chloride, potassium iodide, and iodinated glycerol are not approved by the FDA for use as over-the-counter expectorants. However, they might be found in natural remedies and in prescription medications, and therefore, you need to check the product labels before they are used.

10. Cough Suppressants

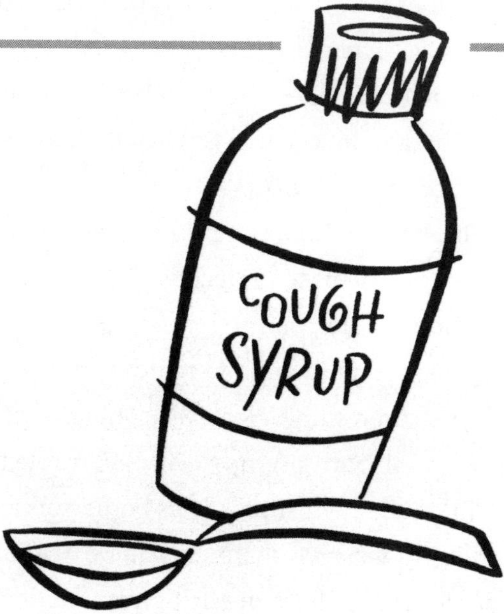

Cough suppressants are a group or class of drugs that are supposed to help relieve or slow down coughing. Some of the FDA recommended ways of describing what these medications may do are: temporarily relieve, calm, control, decrease, or reduce coughing due to minor throat irritation, minor bronchial irritation, or coughing due to the common cold. In medical terms, these drugs are called **antitussives** (tuss means cough–so anti or against coughing).

The U.S. Food and Drug Administration has again made my job in this chapter a little easier. Several years ago, there were many drugs listed as cough suppressants. However, now only six are currently approved for use in this category. Four of these come as an oral medication and two are topical (medicated rubs and/or cough drops). In addition, one of these was fully discussed in the chapter on antihistamines (Chapter 8) and another may no longer be marketed (I can no longer find it where I live). Therefore, the usual sections on warnings, drug interactions, and side effects will be covered under the individual drugs. There is, however, a Crux of the Matter section which is mainly for history buffs.

Finally, coughing is a normal reflex of our body and in many ways it helps to protect us. Therefore, **not all coughing is bad**. If food, water, or another foreign object gets into our airway, we cough in order to remove these materials so normal breathing can resume. However, some things in life (like cold viruses and flu viruses) may actually irritate the throat and bronchial tubes which promotes bothersome coughing. This is where using these medicines might be helpful. In addition, coughing is sometimes the first symptom of a more serious problem involving the heart or lungs. Therefore, if you are using a cough suppressant and your cough is not improving or is becoming worse, you should see your healthcare provider.

The Bottom Line

The current active ingredient list of available cough suppressants found in over-the-counter medications is as follows:

1. Dextromethorphan - pills
2. Codeine - pills
3. Diphenhydramine - pills
4. Chlophedianol - pills
5. Camphor - topical
6. Menthol - topical (cough drops, lozenges)

If my wife were pregnant and she and I and our doctor decided to use a cough suppressant during the pregnancy, I would choose No. 1 (and possibly No. 3). Number 3 was one of the first choices for antihistamines, but there is some question on how well it works as a cough suppressant when compared to number 1 in the list above. If No. 3 is effective for you, then it would also be a good selection. Finally, No. 2 is not all that bad. However, you should read the section on codeine because it can be habit-forming (addicting).

The Crux Of The Matter

The first group of drugs discovered to decrease or minimize coughing were the **narcotics**. Essentially, these medications can only be obtained with a prescription or administered in a hospital. Narcotic drugs are also called **opiates** (named after **opium**) and are considered strong pain medicines. The effects of opium have been known for thousands of years, and unfortunately the drug has been abused by people because of its ability to produce euphoria. In other words, it made people feel good.

The word opium is actually Greek and means juice. Opium is the juice of the poppy seed. The main drug of opium is actually morphine, and this active ingredient was first isolated by a researcher in the early 1800s. He named it after Morpheus, the Greek God of Dreams. Over the next 100 to 150 years, many other drugs related to morphine were discovered or manufactured and today many different narcotic medications are available. Codeine was isolated in the 1830s. Other narcotic drug names you may have heard include heroin (a commonly abused drug), meperidine (marketed as Demerol), oxycodone (marketed as Percodan) and propoxyphene (marketed as

Darvon). Another strong narcotic drug is called Levorphanol (leev-ORF-an-all) which is related to dextromethorphan, but this is discussed in more detail under Dextromethorphan, the first drug on our list.

It was initially determined that narcotic drugs could relieve pain which is their main use today. However, during studies, it was also discovered that these medications could decrease coughing. Unfortunately, the narcotic drugs are habit-forming and many people become addicted to them. Over the years, researchers have tried to develop non-addicting drugs that can suppress coughing. A few non-narcotic cough suppressants are available; however, most of these are still prescription drugs.

1. Dextromethorphan

Dextromethorphan (dex-tro-METH-or-fan) is one of the FDA approved over-the-counter cough suppressants. If you read a label from an OTC cold medication that has the word dextromethorphan (only), dextromethorphan hydrobromide, dextromethorphan HBr, or dextromethorphan polistirex, these essentially mean the same thing. A common brand name (trade name) drug that contains this active ingredient is Delsym; however, numerous OTC products contain dextromethorphan. A common way for stating that a cold remedy contains this active ingredient is with the initials D or DM, such as Robitussin-DM or Triaminic-DM. Please remember, that the active ingredients in a brand name product can change over time. Therefore, you still need to read the labels.

This drug is the **mirror image** of a strong pain medication (narcotic) called levorphanol. The subject of mirror image drugs was discussed in the decongestant chapter under the heading Levmetamfetamine (pages 133-134). Levorphanol is the levo drug. It is a strong pain killer and can also be addicting. The **dextro drug is dextromethorphan** and dextromethorphan does NOT do anything for pain and is also NOT addicting. It does, however, work on suppressing a cough. Remember, some mirror image drugs do not have the same strength or even the same actions as their opposites.

Dextromethorphan can make some people sleepy so the user must be careful when taking this with other medications that cause drowsiness (like antihistamines). For the most part, this drug does not affect the heart, blood pressure, or blood sugar. However, people with liver or kidney problems should talk with their doctor before using this drug because the amount taken and the frequency of use may need adjustment.

Drug Interactions

Drug interactions means that if a person were taking some other medication (prescription or over-the-counter) and decided to take this drug, the combination of the two might cause problems. The list below contains many of the drug categories that could react with dextromethorphan.

- MAO inhibitors
- Drugs used to treat depression
- Drugs used to treat other psychological problems
- Quinidine (a drug used for certain heart problems)

Essentially all of the drug groups listed above are obtained by prescription. Therefore, if you are currently taking any drug, you should talk with your healthcare provider before using dextromethorphan.

Using excess amounts of this drug can cause dizziness, blurred vision, mental status changes, and hallucinations (which is seeing things or hearing things that other people do not see or hear). In addition, some people have complained of nausea and vomiting after use (which is a problem with all drugs for some people).

If You Are Pregnant

Dextromethorphan has not been proven to cause major birth defects in humans. From two studies[1,3], a total of 359 pregnant women were identified who took this drug in the first trimester, and no increase in major birth defects was seen over what was expected. In one of these studies[1], there were 580 women who used this drug at some time in their pregnancy (all three trimesters), and no increase in major birth defects was identified. (For statistical information on the number of pregnant women who took this drug in the first trimester compared to other cough suppressants, see Table 3 on page 262.)

Animal studies (involving mammals) during pregnancy on this particular drug were not found. There was one animal study performed on chick embryos that did identify an increase in major birth defects. The drug was placed directly inside the developing egg. This type of animal study is much further removed from human pregnancy. It involved birds, not mammals, and it eliminated the issue of a drug having to cross a placenta because the medication was placed inside the egg in contact with the developing embryo.

Narcotic drugs have been extensively studied in pregnancy and have never been found to cause birth defects. Because dextromethorphan is the mirror image of a narcotic drug, it is unlikely that this active ingredient would cause birth defects for the general pregnant population.

Based on the above information, this drug would be classified according to the pregnancy risk category as a C (see Chapter 4, How is Drug Safety Determined?).

No long-term effects that may show up later in life have been reported with the use of this drug during pregnancy.

One study in pregnant women did show that the drug might be metabolized (broken down) quicker during pregnancy which in theory could mean that the effects may not last as long. However, if you use this drug while pregnant, do not take it more frequently than recommended unless you talk with your healthcare provider first.

Details About Dextromethorphan

- For dosing information, read the package material carefully because all drugs vary on the amount that can be used and the frequency of their use.
- The onset of action (when you might see some response) is usually about 15 to 30 minutes after taking the drug.
- The duration of action (how long the effect might last) is about five to six hours.
- The absorption (how much is taken into the bloodstream) occurs in the intestines and most of an oral dose is absorbed.
- The metabolism of the drug (how the body breaks down the drug) occurs in the liver; however, not all of the drug is metabolized.

- The elimination of the drug (how the body gets rid of it) is accomplished by the kidneys. The kidneys remove it from the body whether it is metabolized or not.
- The half-life of the drug (the amount of time it takes the body to remove half of the drug still circulating in the bloodstream) is about two to four hours.

Breast-feeding

No thorough studies on breast-feeding and this drug have been reported. This drug can probably be found in breast milk. However, the amount of drug and what effect it may have on the baby is unknown.

2. Codeine

Codeine (CO-deen) is (believe it or not) available over-the-counter in many states in the United States and YES, it is one of the FDA approved OTC cough suppressants. However, about one-third of the states in the U.S. do not allow the sale of this drug over-the-counter. Therefore, you would have to check with your local pharmacy to determine whether or not it is available. The amount of codeine in the OTC products for cough suppression is low. If you read a label from an over-the-counter cold medication that has the word codeine (only) or codeine phosphate, these essentially mean the same thing.

Codeine can cause drowsiness so be careful when using this with other drugs that can make you tired (like antihistamines). For the most part, this drug does not affect the heart or blood sugar. Large doses, however, can cause a drop in blood pressure. People with liver or kidney problems should talk with their doctor before using this drug because the amount taken or how frequently it is used may need adjustment. In addition, using codeine for prolonged periods **can cause dependence and addiction**.

Drug Interactions

Drug interactions means that if a person were taking some other medication (prescription or over-the-counter) and decided to take this drug, the combination of the two might cause problems. The list below contains many of the drug categories that could react with codeine.

- Drugs that can make you sleepy (this might include sleeping pills, tranquilizers, drugs that treat depression, MAO inhibitors, sedatives, or drugs used for psychiatric problems)
- Quinidine (a drug used for certain heart problems)
- Antihistamines (because they also cause drowsiness)
- Alcohol

Most of the above drugs (except for alcohol and antihistamines) are prescription drugs. Therefore, if you are taking any medicine (whether it is prescription or not), before using an over-the-counter drug talk to your healthcare provider to be sure there is no conflict.

Using excess amounts of this drug can cause dizziness, blurred vision, mental status changes, passing out, and hallucinations (which is seeing things or hearing things that other people do not see or hear). In addition, some people have complained of nausea and vomiting after use (which is a problem with all drugs for some people). Codeine can also cause constipation.

If You Are Pregnant

Codeine has not been proven to cause major birth defects in humans. This drug has been extensively studied in human pregnancy. From three large studies[1-3] alone, a total of at least 14,787 pregnant women were identified who took this drug in the first trimester, and no increase in major birth defects was seen over what was expected. In two of these studies[1,2], there were 33,981 women who used this drug at some time in their pregnancy (all three trimesters), and no increase in major birth defects was identified. (For statistical information on the number of pregnant women who took this drug in the first trimester compared to other cough suppressants, see Table 3 on page 262.)

On the other hand, a few studies have analyzed a group of pregnancies where a specific birth defect was found and a slightly higher rate of codeine usage was identified. However, these studies most likely represent populations of women with an underlying genetic risk for birth defects and not a random pregnant population. Furthermore, there have been reports of babies going through **withdrawal** after their mothers had used codeine for a long period of time. This is because codeine can be highly addictive for some individuals.

Finally, this drug has been studied in pregnant animals that were given doses larger than those recommended for humans and no harm was identified.

Because of the conflicting information, this drug would be classified according to the pregnancy risk category as a C, and would be classified as a D if used for a long period of time (see Chapter 4, How is Drug Safety Determined?).

Details About Codeine

- For dosing information, read the package material carefully because all drugs vary on the amount that can be used and the frequency of their use.
- The onset of action (when you might see some response) is about one to two hours after taking the drug.
- The duration of action (how long the effect might last) is about four to eight hours.
- The absorption (how much is taken into the bloodstream) occurs in the intestines and most of an oral dose is absorbed.
- The metabolism of the drug (how the body breaks down the drug) occurs in the liver; however, not all of the drug is metabolized.
- The elimination of the drug (how the body gets rid of it) is accomplished by the kidneys. The kidneys remove it from the body whether it is metabolized or not.
- The half-life of the drug (the amount of time it takes the body to remove half of the drug still circulating in the bloodstream) is about two to four hours.

Breast-feeding

No thorough studies on breast-feeding and this drug have been reported. Codeine can be found in breast milk; however, the measured amount in most cases was very small. The American Academy of Pediatrics states that breast-feeding while taking codeine is acceptable at prescribed doses.

3. Diphenhydramine

This active ingredient was fully discussed in the chapter on antihistamines (Chapter 8) and, therefore, you are referred to pages 149-153 for more information. Some studies have questioned how effective diphenhydramine is as a cough suppressant, but at this time, it is listed as one of the approved over-the-counter drugs for cough suppression by the FDA.

4. Chlophedianol

Chlophedianol (clo-fee-DYE-an-all) is a drug approved by the FDA as an over-the-counter cough suppressant. However, very few, if any, OTC products contain this active ingredient. In addition, very little information exists regarding this drug.

It appears that chlophedianol was originally marketed in the early 1960s and is similar to diphenhydramine (No. 3 above). This drug has primarily been a prescription medication. However, it was recently approved by the FDA for over-the-counter use in 1987 through a new drug application (NDA).

In a large study[1] that analyzed many different drugs taken by women during pregnancy, only one case of chlophedianol use was identified and the outcome of that pregnancy is unknown. Furthermore, no significant details on this drug could be obtained regarding onset of action, duration of action, and half-life. The drug is metabolized by the liver and removed from the body by the kidneys. Animal studies during pregnancy on this particular drug were not found. Therefore, this drug would be classified according to the pregnancy risk category as a C (see Chapter 4, How is Drug Safety Determined?).

No thorough studies on breast-feeding and this drug have been reported

5. Camphor

Camphor (KAM-for) is one of the active ingredients that may be found in nasal mists and topical medicated rubs for the neck and chest. This drug is approved by the FDA for cough suppression as a topical agent. These medicated rubs are not to be used orally. The exact action of this drug is not fully known, but it appears to have a mild local anesthetic effect (meaning it partially numbs the area). Therefore, this medication may help block the irritation in the throat that is promoting the cough.

This drug is often combined with menthol. A common brand name (trade name) product that contains this active ingredient is Vicks VapoRub.

If You Are Pregnant

Camphor has not been proven to cause major birth defects in humans. In one study[1], 168 pregnant women were exposed to this drug in the first trimester, and no increase in major birth defects was seen over what was expected. In this same study, 763 women were found to have been exposed to this drug at some time in their pregnancy (all three trimesters), and no increase in major birth defects was identified. Animal studies during pregnancy on this particular drug were not found.

Based on the above information, this drug would be classified according to the pregnancy risk category as a C (see Chapter 4, How is Drug Safety Determined?).

No long-term effects that may show up later in life have been reported with the use of this drug during pregnancy.

There are a few case reports of accidental poisoning with camphor in women who were pregnant, and one of these resulted in a stillbirth. Therefore, products with camphor should not be used excessively during pregnancy. Because this drug can be found in some nasal mists (which can often be partly swallowed), these products should also be used sparingly.

Details about Camphor

This drug is well absorbed into the bloodstream if taken orally. The onset of action is within a few minutes of usage. However, accurate information on duration of action and metabolism were not found. If excessive amounts are used, the main side effects are nausea and vomiting.

Breast-feeding

No thorough studies on breast-feeding and this drug have been reported.

6. Menthol

Menthol (MEN-thal) is one of the active ingredients found in throat lozenges, cough drops, throat sprays, and topical medicated rubs. The exact action of this drug is not fully known, but it appears to have a cool or soothing effect on mucous membranes. This drug, along with camphor, is approved by the FDA for use as a topical cough suppressant.

This topical ingredient is often found in cough drops. Common brand name (trade name) products that contain this active ingredient are Halls Cough Drops and Vicks Cough Drops.

If You Are Pregnant

No significant information was found regarding this drug in human or animal pregnancies. However, menthol has been around for years and is present in many different items taken orally. Based on this information, menthol would be classified according to the pregnancy risk category as a C (see Chapter 4, How is Drug Safety Determined?).

No long-term effects that may show up later in life have been reported with the use of this drug during pregnancy.

Details about Menthol

No accurate information regarding absorption, duration of action, metabolism or elimination were found. If excessive amounts are used, the main side effect is nausea.

Breast-feeding

No thorough studies on breast-feeding and this drug have been reported.

Others

I bet you are now asking—What is an "other"? Well, there are three other non-narcotic drugs that have been developed for use as cough suppressants. It is possible that some time in the future, one or all of these could become over-the-counter medications. Therefore, to be complete, a short discussion on each is included. Because they are non-narcotic medications, they are not addictive or habit forming. The three drugs are benzonatate, carbetapentane, and caramiphen.

Benzonatate (ben-ZOE-na-tate) is currently a prescription medicine used as a cough suppressant. This drug is related to a group of medications called anesthetics which are used for numbing things. In one study[1], only two patients with first trimester exposure were identified, and exact details regarding outcome were not supplied. This drug would be classified as a pregnancy risk category C (see pages 66-67).

Carbetapentane (car-BAY-TA-pen-tane) is also a prescription drug used as a cough suppressant. One of the major side effects seen with this drug is sedation. In other words, it can make you drowsy. Therefore, it would have the same precautions as other sedating drugs. Carbetapentane has been studied in pregnant animals that were given doses larger than those recommended for humans and no harm was identified. No information on first trimester exposure in human pregnancies was found. Therefore, this drug would be classified as a pregnancy risk category C (see pages 66-67).

Finally, **Caramiphen** (ka-RAM-eh-fen) was around for years over-the-counter. However, I can no longer find it and, therefore, it may no longer be manufactured. It is not currently approved by the FDA as an over-the-counter cough suppressant. One study[1] identified 38 women who took this drug in the first trimester, and there was a higher rate of birth defects over what was expected. However, there was no pattern to the birth defects, and 38 patients is a very small number. This same study reported 236 women who used the drug at some time in their pregnancy (all three trimesters), and no increase in major birth defects was identified.

Animal studies during pregnancy on this particular drug were not found. This medication would be classified as a pregnancy risk category C (see pages 66-67).

11. Inactive Ingredients & Other Things

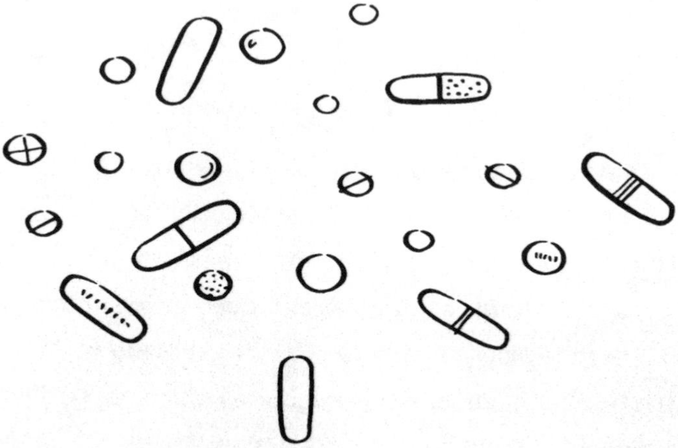

The information contained in this chapter could be very important for pregnant women and also for women who have certain medical conditions such as diabetes. As you will see, some inactive ingredients are not actually inactive—they just don't treat a specific symptom of a cold. Therefore, it is just as important to read the inactive ingredient section (of a drug label or package insert) as it is to read the active ingredient section. Some substances that you might see listed as inactive ingredients include:

1. Sugar
2. Sugar substitutes
3. Alcohol
4. Caffeine
5. Preservatives, lubricants and other things

Sugar, sugar substitutes, and alcohol are usually found in medications that come in liquid form. Two other categories that will be discussed in this chapter are:

6. Pain medications and
7. Drying agents

1. Sugar

Many different sugars can be found in over-the-counter medications. Its purpose is to make the disagreeable taste of a medicine more tolerable. The quantity of sugar in a dose of medication is fairly small, so for most people the amount will not affect the blood sugar level. However, having sugar included could be a problem for some pregnant women, especially if they are diabetic or have developed gestational diabetes.

Furthermore, ALL pregnant women should know that sugar can be found in many over-the-counter medicines. This information is important because blood sugar testing may be performed during the pregnancy. One such test may be a fasting blood sugar level. A fasting blood sugar is usually collected first thing in the morning before eating breakfast, and some people may not think the cold remedy counts because it is not food. However, if the OTC product contains sugar, and the medication is taken before the blood is drawn, it could give a false test result.

Some of the sugars found in OTC cold remedies are **fructose**, **sucrose**, **lactose**, and **glucose**.

2. Sugar Substitutes

The two sugar substitutes, **saccharin** and **aspartame**, may also be present in some OTC medications to help make them taste better. The quantity of sugar substitutes in a given dose of medication is also fairly small, but these substances do not affect the blood sugar level. However, some people may have anxiety about using sugar substitutes.

Saccharin

Saccharin (SACK-rin) has been used in the United States since the early 1900s. Over the years, many concerns about this substance have been voiced. However, no studies have ever documented saccharin as being harmful when used in moderation. Many of the evaluations involving this ingredient focused on its potential for producing cancer. In pregnancy, multiple animal studies were performed using amounts that far exceeded what humans would use and no increase in major birth defects was seen. In addition, no human studies have ever proven that saccharin causes birth defects.

Some organizations state that saccharin should be used with caution during pregnancy, while others feel that its use is safe. The primary purpose of this section is to inform you that saccharin can sometimes be found in OTC drugs. Whether or not this sugar substitute is used is a decision between you and your healthcare provider.

Aspartame

Aspartame (as-SPAR-tame) was discovered in 1965 and approved by the FDA for consumer use in the early 1980s. This substance went through an extensive evaluation by the FDA before it was approved for use by humans. It actually consists of a combination of two amino acids. Twenty amino acids exist in nature and they are the building blocks of our proteins. The two amino acids which make up aspartame are phenylalanine (fen-ul-AL-an-een) and aspartate (as-PAR-tate). In pregnancy, multiple animal studies were performed using amounts that far exceeded what humans would use and no increase in major birth defects was seen. In addition, no human studies have proven that aspartame causes birth defects. Furthermore, because it is made from amino acids (which are part of proteins), it seems logical that this substance would not be a problem for most people when used in moderation.

However, some individuals with a metabolic disorder called PKU (which stands for phenylketonuria) must be very careful with aspartame. People with PKU have a problem breaking down (metabolizing) the amino acid phenylalanine. If a women with PKU is pregnant and her phenylalanine level is too high, her baby could suffer brain damage. Persons with this metabolic problem usually know who they are and should be aware that over-the-counter drugs may contain aspartame. This sugar substitute is not recommended for use by people with PKU. The American Academy of Pediatrics states that aspartame should be used with caution while breast-feeding.

3. Alcohol

Alcohol can also be found in some over-the-counter cold remedies. The amount of alcohol in a dose of medication is usually small. Pregnant women should know that this drug can cause a birth defect called **fetal alcohol syndrome**. This is a severe birth anomaly that produces an unusual looking face, a small head size (microcephally), and mental retardation. The exact relationship between alcohol use and this birth defect are unknown. However, it is most often seen in cases where the mother drank alcoholic beverages throughout the pregnancy.

If a person were to take an over-the-counter medication that contains alcohol and is following the directions, the duration of drug use would only be about 7 to 10 days. This level of exposure has never been proven to cause fetal alcohol syndrome. The purpose for this discussion is to inform pregnant women that alcohol may be found in some OTC drugs so that an educated choice about usage can be made. If alcohol use during pregnancy is considered, you should talk with your healthcare provider first.

4. Caffeine

Caffeine is another substance that is often listed as an inactive ingredient. It may be found in some cold remedies as a "picker upper." Because a cold virus infection may make you tired, and some cold remedies can produce drowsiness, caffeine is added to potentially "pep you up." Caffeine and caffeine-like substances are found in many foods such as coffee, tea, colas, and chocolate.

This drug has been extensively studied in pregnant animals and many reports on human pregnancies also exist. Putting these all together, it appears that caffeine used in moderation is probably not a problem for pregnant women. This ingredient can cross over the placenta to the baby. When consumed in large amounts, a few studies have reported a temporary increase in the baby's heart rate. In most cases, the amount of caffeine in OTC medications is considered small to moderate (equal to about a small cup of coffee).

Again, the purpose of this discussion is to alert you to the fact that caffeine can be listed as an inactive ingredient in some over-the-counter medications.

Caffeine is also available as an OTC medication that can be used when a person feels drowsy but wants to be alert. Common brand name (trade name) products that contain caffeine for this purpose are No Doz and Vivarin. The amount of caffeine in a single dose (200 milligrams) is equivalent to about two cups of coffee.

For those individuals interested in making comparisons, a cup of coffee contains about 65 to 150 milligrams of caffeine, a cup of tea contains about 50 milligrams, a twelve ounce can of a cola drink has about 50 milligrams, and a one ounce chocolate bar contains about 25 milligrams.

5. Preservatives, Lubricants, And Other Things

At one time, I attempted to make an inventory of all the different substances listed as inactive ingredients, but I stopped after passing 150. Besides the active ingredient, sugar, sugar substitutes, alcohol and caffeine, many other substances can be found in OTC products including: preservatives (which keep the medication active), lubricants (which help the medicine slide down the throat easier), colorings, and flavorings. There can also be materials that maintain the shape of the pill while others facilitate the dissolving process once the pill or capsule reaches the stomach.

To sum it up, no adequate information exists about these materials and pregnancy. In general, it seems unlikely that these substances are harmful because many of them are poorly absorbed into the bloodstream. The exact answer to this question, however, is unknown.

6. Pain Medications

It is very common for many OTC cold remedies to also contain a pain medication such as **aspirin**, **acetaminophen**, or **ibuprofen**. These drugs will be fully covered in the next book. They are mentioned here because you should know that they are found in some OTC cold remedies. If you were to take a pain medication in conjunction with a cold remedy (that also contains a pain medication), the double dose could lead to potential problems. For now, aspirin and ibuprofen can be a concern for some women when used during pregnancy. Therefore, acetaminophen is the best choice for treating pain while pregnant, but you should talk with your healthcare provider before use.

7. Drying Agents

The drying agents used to be one of the classes of drugs that could be taken as an over-the-counter cold remedy. The U.S. Food and Drug Administration made my job extremely easy in this case by not approving any for use as OTC drugs. At one time, they were fairly common. The drying agents were supposed to help dry up a runny nose and possibly decrease the amount of mucus made by the lungs. The reason for including this topic in this chapter is that some of these substances may still be found in **natural remedies**. HOWEVER, their use during pregnancy may not be prudent.

The FDA determined that drying agents were probably safe at the doses found in OTC products but did not find them to be effective in doing what they claimed to do. The actual chemical name for the drying agents is **anticholinergics** (anti-COAL-in-er-jiks), a word briefly mentioned in other chapters in this book. The list below contains the names of many of the ingredients (drugs and natural substances) found in this drug category. In addition, many are still found in prescription drugs and can be used for treating stomach problems, intestinal problems, motion sickness, eye problems, and some respiratory disorders. The drug names to look for in natural remedies are as follows:

Atropa belladonna	Belladonna extract
Datura stramonium	Deadly nightshade
Devil's apple	Hyoscyamus niger
Jamestown weed	Jimson weed
Scopolia carniolica	Stink weed
Thorn-apple	Tincture of belladonna
Atropine	Homatropine
Hyoscine	Hyoscyamine
Methscopolamine	Scopolamine

Some of the history behind these drugs and the reason why they could be a problem for pregnancy is discussed further in The Crux of the Matter which follows.

The Crux Of The Matter

The anticholinergic drugs have been around for thousands of years. The original substance came from a plant called the deadly nightshade plant. In the middle ages, this extract was used as a poison. This plant was later named Atropa belladonna. The atropa part was named after Atropos, the oldest of the Three Fates, and the one who cuts the thread of life. This substance was eventually isolated in the early1830s and was called atropine (AT-tro-peen).

Atropine was also found in a plant called Datura stramonium (also called Jamestown weed or Jimson weed). A relative to atropine is scopolamine (sco-PALL-am-meen). Scopolamine can be found in plants called Hyoscyamus niger and Scopolia carniolica.

In a way, belladonna has become a catch-all word for most of the drugs in this category. The belladonna drugs were found to affect the human body in many different places as listed below.

- Brain - causes sleepiness and forgetfulness
- Heart - causes the heart rate to increase
- Intestines - slows down the muscle contractions of the intestines
- Eye - dilates the pupil (makes the dark center part of the eye get larger)
- Skin - stops sweating so the skin becomes dry and hot
- Mouth - dries up the mouth and causes thirst
- Bladder - makes urinating difficult

As you can see, these drugs can affect many parts of the human body. Therefore, they should be used with caution by people who have heart disease, high blood pressure, liver disease, glaucoma (an eye disorder), bladder problems, and chronic lung problems.

For Pregnant Women

These drugs can cross the placenta and potentially affect the baby. Regarding first trimester exposures, several studies have identified women who used these drugs, and no increase in major birth defects was seen over what was expected. Currently, they are classified as category C drugs for use during pregnancy (see Chapter 4, pages 66-67).

However, there are reports of these drugs increasing a baby's heart rate (called tachycardia), and they can also change the way the heart rate looks when recorded on a fetal monitor (it becomes **flatter looking**). This effect on the unborn baby's heart can last for some time. Therefore, these drugs should be used with caution during pregnancy especially in the last trimester (third trimester) of pregnancy.

Two other interesting pieces of information and then I'll stop, I promise. The first is that these drugs might be used to treat mushroom poisoning; however, this should always be done in a hospital. The second is that scopolamine combined with morphine was commonly used to treat labor pain years ago. This therapy was called **twilight sleep**, but this treatment is no longer used today (at least I hope it isn't).

12. Throat Lozenges & Throat Sprays

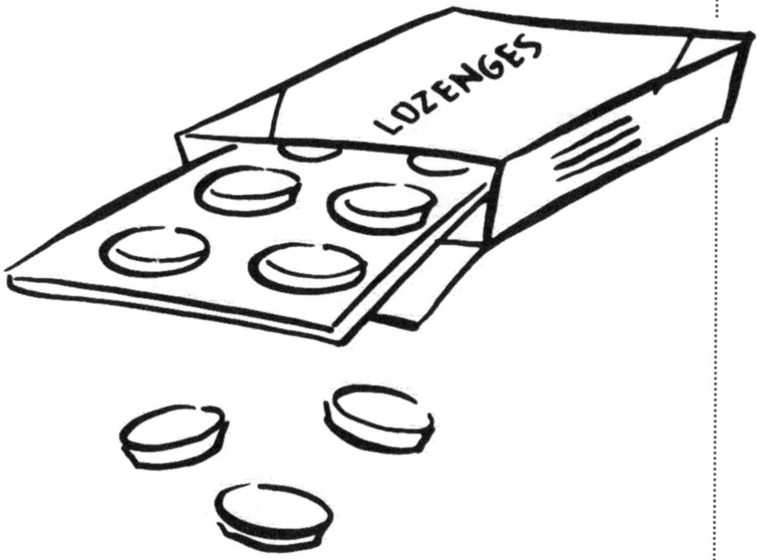

Throat lozenges, cough drops, and throat sprays contain drugs that you should know about. The reason they help soothe a sore throat is because a drug or a chemical is doing something. Throat lozenges and throat sprays are used by most people to help relieve the pain of a sore throat.

Most sore throats are caused by viruses and are often one of the symptoms that go along with a stuffy nose, chest congestion and a cough. A few throat infections can be caused by bacteria (like strep throat). If you have a high fever or a sore throat that lasts for more than two or three days, you should talk with your healthcare provider who may want you to get a throat culture.

Most of the active ingredients that are found in throat lozenges and throat sprays are considered anesthetics, soothing agents, or are antiseptic/disinfectant chemicals. The list below is somewhat organized according to how the medication works.

1. Dyclonine
2. Benzocaine
3. Camphor
4. Menthol
5. Phenol
6. Resorcinol
7. Boric Acid
8. Cetylpyridinium
9. Other Substances

The Bottom Line

To be honest, the majority of the above listed drugs have not been thoroughly studied in human pregnancies, so our knowledge regarding their safety is limited. The discussion on the individual drugs below will cover their mechanism of action, why they are in throat products, and any potential side effects.

Two active ingredients (numbers 2 and 3 above) should be used sparingly during pregnancy because of reported complications from excessive usage. Furthermore, most brand name throat lozenge products are marketed as regular strength and maximum strength, and the active ingredient components are usually different between these two strengths. Therefore, you need to read the labels.

1. Dyclonine

Dyclonine (DYE-klon-neen) is one of the active ingredients found in throat lozenges and throat sprays. This drug is a local **anesthetic** (an-ness-THET-ic), a chemical that causes numbness. For example, if you are cut and need stitches, the doctor in the emergency room will probably numb the area with an anesthetic before he or she puts in the sutures. There are two main categories of anesthetics, esters and amides. Dyclonine is considered an ester anesthetic.

Common brand name (trade name) medications that may contain this active ingredient are Sucrets Throat Lozenges and Cepacol Throat Spray. However, please remember that the active ingredients in a brand name product can change over time. Therefore, you still need to read the labels.

The reason this drug is found in OTC throat lozenges and throat sprays is because it will actually numb the back of the throat where it is hurting. Thus, the sore throat feels better. However, this medication does nothing to cure the problem. If you read a label from an OTC throat lozenge/spray that has the word dyclonine (only), dyclonine hydrochloride, or dyclonine HCl, they essentially mean the same thing.

If You Are Pregnant

Dyclonine has not been proven to cause major birth defects in humans. However, no information on first trimester exposure in human pregnancy was found. In addition, animal studies during pregnancy on this particular drug were not found. This medication is similar to another anesthetic called **procaine** (a drug which is not available over-the-counter). In one study[1], a total of 1,340 women with first trimester exposure to procaine were identified, and no increase in major birth defects was seen over what was expected. In the same study, 3,395 women were exposed to procaine at some time in their pregnancy (all three trimesters), and no increase in major birth defects was identified.

Because no direct information on dyclonine and pregnancy can be found, this drug would be classified according to the pregnancy risk category as a C (see Chapter 4, pages 66-67).

No long-term effects that may show up later in life have been reported with the use of this drug in pregnancy.

Details About Dyclonine

Studies show that the drug is well absorbed into the bloodstream shortly after it is used. The onset of action occurs within a few minutes, and the numbness may last for about 30 minutes. Because this drug is an ester anesthetic, it is metabolized by an enzyme in the bloodstream. If an excessive amount of dyclonine is used, or if a large amount is absorbed, some potential side effects might include nervousness, dizziness, blurred vision, shaky hands, nausea, vomiting, or ringing in the ears.

This medication might make some sulfa antibiotics less effective. Therefore, if you are taking a **sulfa antibiotic**, you should use dyclonine with caution.

Breast-feeding

No thorough studies on breast-feeding and this drug have been reported.

2. Benzocaine

Benzocaine (BEN-zo-kane) is one of the active ingredients found in throat lozenges and throat sprays. This drug is another local anesthetic (see Dyclonine above) and when used, will numb the back of the throat where it is hurting. Again, this drug does nothing to cure the sore throat. If you read a label from an OTC throat lozenge/spray that has the words benzocaine, benzocainum, or ethyl aminobenzoate, they essentially mean the same thing.

Benzocaine is also considered an ester-type anesthetic. Common brand name (trade name) medications that may contain this active ingredient are Vicks Chloraseptic Sore Throat Lozenges and Cepacol Maximum Strength Throat Lozenges. However, please remember that the active ingredients in a brand name product can change over time. Therefore, you still need to read the labels.

If You Are Pregnant

Benzocaine has not been proven to cause major birth defects in humans. In one study[1], 47 pregnant women were exposed to this drug in the first trimester, and no increase in major birth defects was seen over what was expected. In the same study, 238 women were exposed at some time in their pregnancy (all three trimesters), and no increase in major birth defects was identified. Animal studies during pregnancy on this particular drug were not found.

Benzocaine is also similar to another anesthetic called procaine. Information on procaine can be found under Dyclonine (pages 215-216). Because information on benzocaine and pregnancy is limited, this drug would be classified according to the pregnancy risk category as a C (see Chapter 4, pages 66-67).

There are numerous reports of a medical problem called **methemoglobinemia** (METH-uh-mo-GLO-bin-eem-ee-uh) developing after the use of benzocaine. Most of these cases occurred in infants and young children following the use of **excessive** amounts; however, a few cases occurred even after recommended doses were used.

Methemoglobinemia (what a conversation stopper!) is a problem that develops in hemoglobin. Hemoglobin is the iron-containing protein that carries oxygen in red blood cells. Some drugs can change normal hemoglobin into methemoglobin, but methemoglobin cannot carry oxygen. If too much hemoglobin is converted to methemoglobin (a problem called methemoglobinemia), a person's skin will become cyanotic (SYE-an-aut-ik) or blue because the blood has a lower level of oxygen. If the low level of oxygen reaches a critical level and is not corrected, serious damage could occur.

Drug-induced methemoglobinemia could affect a pregnant woman at any time in her pregnancy. For the baby, it is unknown if benzocaine crosses the placenta. Furthermore, the fetus does not really produce a significant amount of hemoglobin until after the first trimester. Therefore, if excessive benzocaine usage were to occur in pregnancy, in theory only, the second and third trimesters would be more critical for the baby.

Benzocaine is found in hundreds of OTC products including topical anesthetic skin creams, hemorrhoid creams, toothache medications, and throat products. Since this drug is commonly used nationwide every day, the chances of developing methemoglobinemia would seem very rare. However, this medication should be used sparingly during pregnancy.

No long-term effects that may show up later in life have been reported with the use of this drug in pregnancy.

Details About Benzocaine

This drug is absorbed fairly well into the bloodstream shortly after its use as a throat product. The onset of action occurs within a few seconds, and the numbness may last for about 15 minutes. Because this drug is an ester anesthetic, it is metabolized by an enzyme in the bloodstream. If an excessive amount of benzocaine is used, or if a large amount is absorbed, some potential side effects might include nervousness, dizziness, blurred vision, shaky hands, nausea, vomiting, ringing in the ears, and methemoglobinemia.

This medication might make some sulfa antibiotics less effective. Therefore, if you are taking a **sulfa antibiotic**, you should use benzocaine with caution.

Breast-feeding

No thorough studies on breast-feeding and this drug have been reported.

3. Camphor

Camphor (KAM-for) is one of the active ingredients that may be found in throat lozenges and throat sprays. This drug is usually found in topical medicated rubs. The exact action of this drug is not known. It is not an anesthetic (like dyclonine or benzocaine); however, it appears to have mild local anesthetic properties. Therefore, it may help to numb the back of the throat where it is hurting. The amount of this drug contained in oral products is minimal.

Camphor (along with menthol) is approved by the FDA as a topical agent for use as a cough suppressant. This drug was discussed in detail in Chapter 10 (pages 199-200), and should also be used sparingly during pregnancy.

4. Menthol

Menthol (MEN-thal) is one of the active ingredients found in throat lozenges and throat sprays. The exact action of this drug is not fully known, but it appears to have a cool or soothing effect on mucous membranes. This drug (along with camphor) is approved by the FDA as a topical agent for use as a cough suppressant. Therefore, this drug was discussed in detail in Chapter 10 (pages 200-201).

Common brand name (trade name) medications that may contain this active ingredient are Halls Throat Drops and Cepacol Throat Lozenges. However, please remember that the active ingredients in a brand name product can change over time. Therefore, you still need to read the labels.

5. Phenol

Phenol (FEE-nall) is one of the active ingredients found in throat lozenges and throat sprays. The drug is not an anesthetic (like dyclonine or benzocaine), however, it has topical anesthetic properties. Therefore, it will numb the back of the throat where it is hurting. Phenol is also an antiseptic and disinfectant meaning it may kill bacteria or stop them from growing. This effect might prevent an overgrowth of bacteria during a viral infection. Again, this drug does nothing to cure the sore throat.

If you read a label from an OTC throat lozenge/spray that has the word phenol or carbolic acid, they essentially mean the same thing. A common brand name (trade name) medication that may contain this active ingredient is Vicks Chloraseptic Throat Spray. However, please remember that the active ingredients in a brand name product can change over time. Therefore, you still need to read the labels.

If You Are Pregnant

Phenol has not been proven to cause major birth defects in humans. In one study[1], 23 pregnant women were exposed to this drug in the first trimester, and no increase in major birth defects was seen over what was expected. Animal studies during pregnancy on this particular drug were not found.

Based on the above information, this drug would be classified according to the pregnancy risk category as a C (see Chapter 4, pages 66-67).

No long-term effects that may show up later in life have been reported with the use of this drug in pregnancy.

Details About Phenol

This drug is well absorbed into the bloodstream following its use as a throat product. The onset of action occurs within a few minutes. Significant details on duration of action and metabolism were not obtained. If an excessive amount of drug is used or if a large amount is absorbed, there have been reports of severe drops in blood pressure accompanied by breathing problems. The amount of phenol contained in throat products is minimal. Therefore, this complication is unlikely to occur if the medication is used as directed.

Breast-feeding

No thorough studies on breast-feeding and this drug have been reported.

6. Resorcinol

Resorcinol (re-SOR-sin-nall) is one of the active ingredients found in throat lozenges and throat sprays. This drug is a topical antiseptic and disinfectant. The exact reason this medication is found in OTC throat lozenges and throat sprays is not clear other than it might prevent an overgrowth of bacteria. Again, this drug does nothing to cure the sore throat.

If you read a label from an OTC throat lozenge that has the word resorcinol or hexylresorcinol, they essentially mean the same thing. A common brand name (trade name) medication that may contain this active ingredient is Sucrets Throat Lozenge. However, please remember that the active ingredients in a brand name product can change over time. Therefore, you still need to read the labels.

If You Are Pregnant

Resorcinol has not been proven to cause major birth defects in humans. In one study[1], 8 pregnant women were exposed to this drug in the first trimester, but exact details regarding outcome were not supplied. In the same study, 118 women were exposed to this drug at some time in their pregnancy (all three trimesters), and no increase in major birth defects was identified. Animal studies during pregnancy on this particular drug were not found.

Based on the above information, this drug would be classified according to the pregnancy risk category as a C (see Chapter 4, pages 66-67).

No long-term effects that may show up later in life have been reported with the use of this drug in pregnancy.

Details About Resorcinol

This drug can be absorbed into the bloodstream following its use, and the onset of action occurs within a few minutes. However, significant details on duration of action and metabolism were not found.

Breast-feeding

No thorough studies on breast-feeding and this drug have been reported.

7. Boric Acid

Boric acid is one of the active ingredients that might be found in throat lozenges and throat sprays. This drug is also found in some eye medications because in a liquid form, it is not irritating to the surface of the eye. This medication is considered a topical antiseptic and disinfectant. The exact reason boric acid is found in throat and/or eye products is not completely certain other than it might prevent an overgrowth of bacteria. In addition, this drug does nothing to cure a sore throat.

If You Are Pregnant

Boric acid has not been proven to cause major birth defects in humans. In one study[1], a total of 253 pregnant women were exposed to this drug in the first trimester, and no increase in major birth defects was seen over what was expected. In this same study, 463 women were exposed at some time in their pregnancy (all three trimesters), and no increase in major birth defects was identified. Animal studies during pregnancy on this particular medication were not found.

Based on the above information, this drug would be classified according to the pregnancy risk category as a C (see Chapter 4, pages 66-67).

No long-term effects that may show up later in life have been reported with the use of this drug in pregnancy.

Details About Boric Acid

This drug is well absorbed into the bloodstream whether it is used as a throat product or an eye medication. The onset of action occurs within a few minutes of use, but significant details on duration of action and metabolism were not obtained. If an excessive amount of drug is used or if a large amount is absorbed, there have been reports of nausea, vomiting, diarrhea, and even severe drops in blood pressure accompanied by breathing problems. The amount of boric acid contained in OTC products is minimal. Therefore, this complication is unlikely to occur if the medication is used as directed.

Breast-feeding

No thorough studies on breast-feeding and this drug have been reported.

8. Cetylpyridinium

Cetylpyridinium (see-tul-peer-uh-DIN-ee-um) is one of the active ingredients that might be found in throat lozenges and throat sprays. If you read a label from a throat lozenge/spray product that has the word cetylpyridinium (only) or cetylpyridinium chloride, they essentially mean the same thing. This drug is also considered a topical antiseptic and disinfectant. The exact reason this medication is found in throat products is not completely clear other than it might prevent an overgrowth of bacteria. Cetylpyridinium does nothing to cure the sore throat.

Common brand name (trade name) medications that may contain this active ingredient are Cepacol Throat Lozenges and Cepacol Throat Spray. However, please remember that the active ingredients in a brand name product can change over time. Therefore, you still need to read the labels.

If You Are Pregnant

Cetylpyridinium has not been proven to cause major birth defects in humans. From two studies[1,3], a total of 932 pregnant women were identified who used this drug in the first trimester, and no increase in major birth defects was seen over what was expected. In one of these studies[1], 490 women were exposed to the drug at some time in their pregnancy (all three trimesters), and no increase in major birth defects was identified. Animal studies during pregnancy on this particular medication were not found.

Based on the above information, this drug would be classified according to the pregnancy risk category as a C (see Chapter 4, pages 66-67).

No long-term effects that may show up later in life have been reported with the use of this drug in pregnancy.

Details About Cetylpyridinium

This drug is well absorbed into the bloodstream following its use as a throat product. The onset of action occurs within a few minutes, but significant details on duration of action and metabolism were not obtained. If an excessive amount of drug is used or if a large amount is absorbed, there have been reports of nausea, vomiting, and diarrhea.

Breast-feeding

No thorough studies on breast-feeding and this drug have been reported.

9. Other Substances

Many other substances are found in throat lozenges and throat sprays including sugars, starches, lubricants, stabilizers, colors, flavors, and preservatives. Some of the chemical names you may read are sorbitol, sucrose, citric acid, glycerin, eucalyptus oil, eucalyptol, sodium benzoate, pectin, tartaric acid, sodium citrate, mineral oil, silicon dioxide, antifoam emulsion, gum crystal, phosphoric acid and polysorbate.

Although usually considered an inactive ingredient, **pectin** is listed as an active ingredient in some OTC throat medications. Pectin is not actually absorbed into the bloodstream (similar to sorbitol and glycerin). Its purpose is to add moisture to the affected area and may help soothe a dry scratchy throat. No information was found regarding the use of pectin, sorbitol, or glycerin in pregnancy. Since they are not absorbed, they probably would not be considered a problem for use during pregnancy.

13. Over-The-Counter Drugs For The Eyes

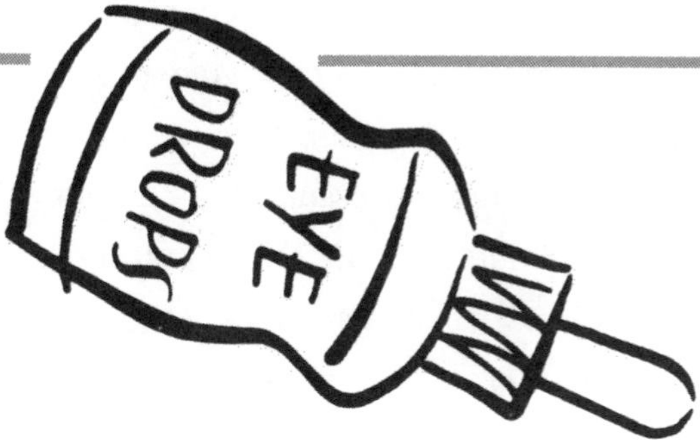

The reason for including this group of drugs is that many people with colds or allergies may also have itchy, watery, irritated eyes. In addition, many of the drugs found in eye products are similar to or are the same as drugs listed in Chapters 7, 8, and 11. Furthermore, the eye is considered a mucous membrane (just like the inside of the nose or mouth), and drugs can be absorbed into the bloodstream. The amount of drug that is absorbed varies from person to person.

The purpose of this chapter is to discuss the active ingredients that might be found in OTC eye products. The available medications can be categorized into drug classifications seen below.

A. Decongestants

B. Antihistamines

C. Belladonna drugs (in natural remedies)

D. Astringents

E. Other things

A. Decongestants

Many OTC eye medicines will contain decongestant-type drugs because they can treat red, irritated eyes by constricting blood vessels. The most common active agents in this group are **naphazoline**, **oxymetazoline**, **phenylephrine**, and **tetrahydrozoline**. Naphazoline, oxymetazoline, and phenylephrine were fully discussed in Chapter 7, Decongestants, and you should return to that chapter for more information about those three active ingredients (pages 106-124).

A common brand name (trade name) product that may contain oxymetazoline is Long Lasting Relief Visine. A common brand name medication that may contain naphazoline is OcuHist. However, remember that the active ingredients in a brand name product can change over time. Therefore, you still need to read the labels.

Information about tetrahydrozoline is found below but as you will see, this drug is very similar to oxymetazoline and naphazoline. Before continuing, if you plan on using an OTC eye medication that has one of the four active ingredients listed above, PLEASE read the sections on Warnings, Drug Interactions, and the Two Sides of Side Effects in Chapter 7 (pages 88-94).

Tetrahydrozoline

Tetrahydrozoline (tet-ruh-hye-DRAW-zo-leen) is a decongestant-type drug that can be found in over-the-counter eye medications. If you read a label from an OTC product for your eyes that has the word tetrahydrozoline (only), tetrahydrozoline hydrochloride, or tetrahydrozoline HCl, they essentially mean the same thing. A common brand name (trade name) medication that may contain this active ingredient is Visine. However, remember that the active ingredients in a brand name product can change over time. Therefore, you still need to read the labels.

When researching this drug, I came across several references that indicated this medicine might also be found in nasal sprays. However, according to the U.S. Food and Drug Administration, it currently is not approved for use as an over-the-counter nasal spray. Therefore, at this time, you can probably only find this drug in OTC eye products.

Sometimes with a cold or the flu (or with allergies or other irritating substance like smoke or dust), your eyes may become irritated and you may see several dilated red blood vessels on the surface of the eyeball. This medication works by constricting those blood vessels (the vessels become smaller). However, you should know that this effect on the eye is only temporary and is not a cure for what is irritating the eyes.

As stated before, tetrahydrozoline is very similar to two other available eye decongestants, oxymetazoline and naphazoline. Tetrahydrozoline is considered a short-acting decongestant drug like naphazoline when compared to other decongestants.

If You Are Pregnant

Tetrahydrozoline has not been proven to cause major birth defects in humans. Only three pregnant women were identified in one study[1] who used this drug in the first trimester, and exact details regarding outcome were not supplied. Please read the section on gastroschisis found on page 98. (For statistical information on the number of pregnant women who used this drug in the first trimester compared to other decongestant-type medications, see Table 1 on page 260.) Animal studies during pregnancy on this particular drug were not found.

Based on the above information, this drug would be classified according to the pregnancy risk category as a C (see Chapter 4, How is Drug Safety Determined?).

No long-term effects that may show up later in life have been reported with the use of this drug during pregnancy.

Tetrahydrozoline (like oxymetazoline) is a fairly potent alpha agent (described on pages 99-106). It has very little beta effect, if any. This means that tetrahydrozoline could constrict blood vessels throughout the body, could raise blood pressure, and might cause uterine contractions (see pages 107-108 under Oxymetazoline). Again, **before you use** tetrahydrozoline or any other decongestant, you must find out if you have toxemia (high blood pressure during pregnancy) and this condition was discussed in more detail on page 89.

Many decongestants can stimulate the brain causing a feeling of being awake or nervous. An interesting finding with tetrahydrozoline is that it may also cause a depressed feeling.

Details About Tetrahydrozoline

- For dosing information, read the package material carefully because all drugs vary on the amount that can be used and the frequency of their use.
- The onset of action (when you can expect some response) is within five minutes of using the medicine.
- The duration of action (how long the effect might last) is two to four hours or longer.
- The absorption (how much is taken into the bloodstream) varies from person to person. The amount of drug absorbed

from the surface of the eye is quite different from drugs absorbed in the intestines. However, tetrahydrozoline can be found in the bloodstream after usage.

- The metabolism of the drug (how the body breaks down the drug) occurs in the liver; however, not all of the drug is metabolized.
- The elimination of the drug (how the body gets rid of it) is accomplished by the kidneys. The kidneys remove it from the body whether it is metabolized or not.
- The half-life of the drug (the amount of time it takes the body to remove half of the drug still circulating in the bloodstream) is about three to six hours.

Breast-feeding

No studies were found involving the use of this drug while breast-feeding. Some studies have looked at other alpha drugs which, if absorbed into the bloodstream, may be found in breast milk. However, in most cases, the amount of the alpha drugs found in breast milk was so small that any effect on the baby would most likely be unnoticed. This is especially true if recommended doses are used. In theory only, if larger than recommended doses were used, some irritability in the baby could be expected.

B. Antihistamines

Some of the OTC eye medications will contain antihistamine-type drugs because the eyes can become red and irritated due to allergy-type reactions. The most common active ingredient in this drug category is **pheniramine**. Another available antihistamine is **antazoline** (see below). Pheniramine was fully discussed in Chapter 8, Antihistamines (page 166).

Common brand name (trade name) medications that may contain pheniramine are OcuHist and Naphcon. However, remember that the active ingredients in a brand name product can change over time. Therefore, you still need to read the labels.

Again, if you plan to use an OTC eye medication that has an antihistamine, PLEASE read the sections on Warnings, Drug Interactions, and the Two Sides of Side Effects in Chapter 8.

Antazoline

Antazoline is another antihistamine that may be found in OTC eye medications. This drug was approved for over-the-counter use in 1994 under a new drug application. If you read a label from an OTC product for the eyes that has the word antazoline (only) or antazoline phosphate, they essentially mean the same thing. A listed brand name (trade name) medication that may contain this active ingredient is Vasocon. However, remember that the active ingredients in a brand name product can change over time. Therefore, you still need to read the labels.

This antihistamine is similar to pheniramine and is an H-1 blocking agent. Therefore, the same precautions regarding drowsiness should be taken. This ingredient is often combined with naphazoline (a decongestant drug).

If You Are Pregnant

Antazoline has not been proven to cause major birth defects in humans. However, no information on first trimester exposure in human pregnancy was found. In addition, animal studies during pregnancy on this particular drug were not found.

Because the information on antazoline and pregnancy is limited, this drug would be classified according to the pregnancy risk category as a C (see Chapter 4, How is Drug Safety Determined?).

Details About Antazoline

No significant details on this drug could be obtained regarding onset of action, duration of action, and half-life. The drug is probably metabolized by the liver, and the kidneys probably eliminate it from the body whether it is metabolized or not.

Breast-feeding

No thorough studies on breast-feeding and this drug have been reported. Antazoline can probably be found in breast milk. However, the amount of drug and what effect it may have on the baby is unknown.

C. Belladonna Drugs

Belladonna drugs are also called **anticholinergic** medications, and this subject was fully discussed in Chapter 11, pages 209-212. Anticholinergic drugs are not approved by the FDA for use as over-the-counter medicines. The purpose for mentioning them here is that they may be found in natural remedies, and anticholinergic medications can affect a pregnancy. Therefore, if you plan to use an OTC natural product for the eye that contains a belladonna ingredient, please be sure to read the section in Chapter 11 first.

D. Astringents

By definition, an astringent draws or pulls things together, and the most common astringent found in eye medications is zinc sulfate. This ingredient promotes the release of protein which helps clear mucus from the surface of the eye. This process eases the itching and burning. No information on zinc sulfate and its use during pregnancy was found. However, zinc is a mineral needed by the body and is considered a pregnancy risk category A substance when consumed in amounts suggested by the recommended daily allowance (RDA).

Zinc can inhibit the absorption of copper, and copper is another mineral the body needs. If large amounts of zinc are used and absorbed, a copper deficiency could develop. In addition, anemia (low red blood cell count), nausea, and vomiting have been reported with excessive zinc consumption. Individuals with glaucoma should talk with their healthcare provider prior to using zinc sulfate or any astringent.

E. Other Things

The other things that may be found in OTC eye medicines are substances or chemicals that help moisturize the eye if it is dry. These ingredients may also be preservatives or antiseptics and disinfectants. Again, very little information about these substances in pregnancy can be found. However, most of them are poorly absorbed and probably only work locally. Some words you may see include glycerin, glycerol, sodium chloride, boric acid, povidone, polyvinyl alcohol, sorbitol, polyethylene glycol, eucalyptol, and sodium phosphate, to name a few. Boric acid was discussed in detail in Chapter 12 (page 223).

14. Medicines For Asthma & Allergy Prevention

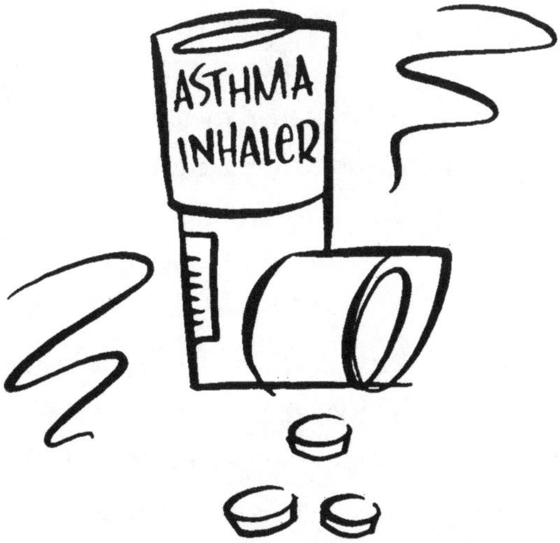

This chapter briefly discusses the drugs found over-the-counter for treating asthma and preventing respiratory allergies. Very few drugs are available for these disorders because most of the medications require a prescription. Currently there are two for asthma, and both are similar to the decongestant drugs. Thus, it seemed appropriate to include them in this book.

Asthma is a very common disease. Some estimates claim that 5 out of every 100 people in the United States have some form of asthma meaning millions of people suffer from this condition. About half of the asthmatics (people with asthma) are children under the age of ten, and it is more common in boys (approximately two boys for every girl). Furthermore, asthma is a very common medical disorder seen in pregnant women.

In short, asthma is a disease where a person's breathing passageways become narrow (the small tubes or spaces inside the lungs become smaller) making it difficult to breathe. A variety of drugs are available for treating this problem, but most of them are by prescription only.

This disease is unusual because most people with asthma are not constantly short of breath. At times they seem perfectly fine, and then all of a sudden they develop an **asthma attack**. When a person has an asthma attack, you may hear high pitched breathing sounds (wheezing) when they exhale. An extensive amount of research has been conducted in an effort to identify the factors that induce these attacks. The more common causes identified are allergic reactions, drug reactions, infections, exercise, and emotional stresses.

Allergic reactions may be caused by substances in the environment such as pollens or dust as well as occupational exposures (chemicals). The list of possible drugs that might bring on an asthma attack is nearly endless. However, one important drug to mention is **aspirin** which is a problem for many asthmatics. Infections can also trigger an asthma attack. Under this category, viruses are a common culprit (especially cold and flu viruses). Finally, some people can develop asthma attacks because of strenuous exercise or emotional stress.

Down To Two

A few years ago, there were three available drugs that could be purchased over-the-counter for treating asthma. They were theophylline, epinephrine, and ephedrine. The FDA removed theophylline from the list as an OTC drug, so now there are two.

These two drugs still cause concern because of potential abuse and, therefore, may be removed sometime in the future. There are many arguments about this topic. Some believe that they should be available over-the-counter because of the enormous number of people who suffer from asthma. Others argue that these two drugs are very powerful, and people with asthma should be monitored by someone in the healthcare profession.

For those of you with asthma, if an asthma attack develops during a pregnancy, PLEASE talk to your obstetrical caregiver **before you use** any over-the-counter drug for treatment. Asthma in pregnancy can affect the baby in many ways and your doctor or healthcare provider needs to know when an attack is occurring. This is especially true for those women in the last trimester of a pregnancy because, based on the severity of the attack, fetal monitoring for the baby may be indicated.

The two available drugs currently found over-the-counter for treating asthma and a third drug which is available for preventing respiratory allergies are listed below.

1. Epinephrine (asthma)
2. Ephedrine (asthma)
3. Cromolyn sodium (respiratory allergy prevention)

1. Epinephrine

Epinephrine (EP-uh-NEF-rin) is commonly known as adrenaline and has many different uses in the field of medicine. If you are pregnant, you must talk with your healthcare provider before using this medication. This drug was briefly discussed in the section called The Crux of the Matter in Chapter 7 (page 99). Epinephrine can only be found over-the-counter as an inhaler. It is not available in pill form at the present time.

A common brand name (trade name) medication that contains this active ingredient is Primatene Mist. However, remember that the active ingredients in a brand name product can change over time. Therefore, you still need to read the labels.

This drug works by dilating the smooth muscles inside the lungs. This allows a person to breathe easier. All of the **Warnings**, **Drug Interactions** and **Side Effects** for this drug are the same as those seen for decongestants (see Chapter 7, pages 88-94).

If You Are Pregnant

Epinephrine has not actually been proven to cause major birth defects in humans. In one study[1], a total of 189 pregnant women were identified who used epinephrine in the first trimester and an **increase** in overall birth defects was seen over what was expected, but there was **no pattern** to the defects. In a second study[2], there were 35 women with first trimester exposure, and no increase in major birth defects was identified. From both of these studies[1,2], there were a total of 636 women who used this drug at some time in their pregnancy (all three trimesters), and no increase in major birth defects was found. (For statistical information on the number of pregnant women who took this drug in the first trimester compared to similar drugs, see Table 1 on page 260.) Animal studies during pregnancy have been performed and an **increase** in birth defects was seen when doses **25 times larger** than a human dose were given.

Because of the above conflicting information, this drug would be classified according to the pregnancy risk category as a C (see Chapter 4, pages 66-67).

Epinephrine has both an alpha effect and a beta effect (discussed on pages 99-106). Its alpha effect is very strong and it can have a tremendous effect on the heart as well as blood pressure (by constricting blood vessels). If taken in large doses, it could slow down blood flow to the uterus. Therefore, epinephrine should only be used in pregnancy **after** consulting your health-care provider. This is especially true if you have hypertension or toxemia (high blood pressure during pregnancy).

Its action upon the muscles of the uterus is unknown. The alpha effect would promote contractions, but the beta effect would cause relaxation.

Details About Epinephrine

For dosing information, read the package material carefully because all drugs vary on the amount that can be used and the frequency of their use. The onset of action is usually within a few minutes; however, no significant details on this drug could be obtained regarding duration of action or half-life. The drug is rapidly metabolized in the liver.

Breast-feeding

No thorough studies on breast-feeding and this drug have been reported. Epinephrine can probably be found in breast milk. However, the amount of drug and what effect it may have on the baby is unknown.

2. Ephedrine

Ephedrine (ef-FED-rin) is usually found over-the-counter in pill form. If you are pregnant, **you must talk** with your healthcare provider before using this medication. All of the **Warnings**, **Drug Interactions** and **Side Effects** for this drug are the same as those seen for decongestants (see Chapter 7, pages 88-94).

A common brand name (trade name) medication that contains this active ingredient is Primatene Tablets. However, please remember that the active ingredients in a brand name product can change over time. Therefore, you still need to read the labels. Primatene Tablets are a prime example of this concept. This brand name used to contain theophylline and ephedrine before theophylline was removed from an OTC status.

One of the FDA's concerns about ephedrine is that sometimes people use it to make illegal drugs such as **methamphetamine** (METH-am-FET-uh-meen). For this reason, ephedrine may eventually be removed from OTC drug products. Ephedrine is another ingredient that can be found in over-the-counter **natural remedies** and these **should be avoided** during pregnancy.

If You Are Pregnant

Ephedrine has not been proven to cause major birth defects in humans. From two studies[1,2], a total of 469 pregnant women were identified who used this drug in the first trimester, and no increase in major birth defects was seen over what was expected. In one of these studies[1], there were 873 women who used this drug at some time in their pregnancy (all three trimesters), and no increase in major birth defects was identified. Please read the section on gastroschisis found on page 98. (For statistical information on the number of pregnant women who took this drug in the first trimester compared to similar drugs, see Table 1 on page 260.) Animal studies during pregnancy on this particular drug were not found.

Despite the above information, this drug would still be classified according to the pregnancy risk category as a C (see Chapter 4, pages 66-67).

No long-term effects that may show up later in life have been reported with the use of this drug during pregnancy.

Ephedrine has both an alpha and a beta effect similar to pseudoephedrine (a decongestant drug, see pages 99-106.) Because it has an alpha effect, it might constrict blood vessels throughout the body which could lead to an increase in blood pressure. Again, **before you use** ephedrine, you must find out if you have toxemia (high blood pressure during pregnancy).

The fact that ephedrine has an alpha effect also means that it could lead to contractions in the uterus, HOWEVER, since this drug also has a **beta effect** this would tend to relax the uterus. The question of uterine contractions and ephedrine has not been thoroughly studied. However, based on the fact that muscles of the uterus relax when exposed to beta drugs, there probably would be either no effect on the uterus or the uterus would tend to relax if exposed to this drug.

Details About Ephedrine

- For dosing information, read the package material carefully because all drugs vary on the amount that can be used and the frequency of their use.
- The onset of action (when you can expect some response) is within five to ten minutes of using the medicine.
- The duration of action (how long the effect might last) is about two hours.
- The absorption (how much is taken into the bloodstream) occurs in the intestines, and most of an oral dose is absorbed.
- The metabolism of the drug (how the body breaks down the drug) occurs in the liver; however, only a small amount is broken down. The rest of the drug remains unchanged in the bloodstream until it is eliminated.
- The elimination of the drug (how the body gets rid of it) is accomplished by the kidneys. The kidneys remove it from the body whether it is metabolized or not.
- The half-life of the drug (the amount of time it takes the body to remove half of the drug still circulating in the bloodstream) is about three to six hours.

Breast-feeding

No thorough studies on breast-feeding and this drug have been reported. There is one report of a baby that became irritable with a lot of crying and sleep problems when the mother used a cold medicine that contained ephedrine with an antihistamine. When the mother stopped the drug, the symptoms in the baby improved. In most cases, if used as recommended, there would be little effect seen in a nursing child.

3. Cromolyn Sodium

Cromolyn (CHROME-o-lin) sodium is the third drug to be discussed in this chapter. This is an over-the-counter medication which can be used to prevent respiratory allergies. This drug used to be a prescription medication but was approved by the FDA for over-the-counter use in 1997. Cromolyn sodium is only available as a nasal inhaler. A common brand name (trade name) medication that contains this active ingredient is Nasalcrom. However, remember that the active ingredients in a brand name product can change over time. Therefore, you still need to read the labels.

This drug was synthesized in the mid-1960s and has been used for treating respiratory allergies and asthma since the mid-1970s. It works by preventing the release of histamine by certain cells in the body. (Histamine was discussed in detail in Chapter 8, Antihistamines, pages 145-147.) This action is different from the antihistamines (which can only block the effects of histamine after it has been released). For people who suffer from respiratory allergies, the primary use of this drug is prevention. Therefore, if possible, it should be used prior to being exposed to the irritating substance.

This drug is poorly absorbed into the bloodstream, so drug interactions are rare. In addition, this medication has few side effects. When used in large amounts, some of the observed side effects include drowsiness, headache, nausea, mental confusion, and nasal burning. There are rare individuals who actually develop sneezing and shortness of breath (an opposite reaction) after using this inhaler. These individuals are probably allergic to cromolyn sodium.

If You Are Pregnant

Cromolyn sodium has not been proven to cause major birth defects in humans. In one study[2], a total of 191 pregnant women were identified who used this drug in the first trimester, and no increase in major birth defects was seen over what was expected. In the same study, there were 488 women who used this drug at some time in their pregnancy (all three trimesters), and no increase in major birth defects was found. A second study identified 296 women who used the drug throughout pregnancy and again, no increase in major birth defects was seen over what was expected. This drug has also been studied in pregnant animals that were given doses much larger than those recommended for humans and no harmful effects were identified.

The manufacturer has listed this drug as category B. I would also classify cromolyn sodium as a pregnancy risk category B (see Chapter 4, pages 66-67) because very little of the drug is absorbed into the bloodstream. There is also a question about whether the drug can even cross the placenta. Therefore, exposure to the unborn baby would be extremely minimal, especially if the medication is used as directed.

It is important to recognize that most individuals who suffer from respiratory allergies may use this medication for several weeks at a time during the "allergy season." If you are pregnant and have respiratory allergies, you should still speak with your healthcare provider before using this medication.

Details About Cromolyn Sodium

- For dosing information, read the package material carefully because all drugs vary on the amount that can be used and the frequency of their use.
- The onset of action (when you might see some response) is usually within a few minutes of use.
- The duration of action (how long the effect might last) varies from person to person. After extended use, the prevention quality of the drug can last for days.
- The absorption (how much is taken into the bloodstream) of this drug is poor. Less than 10 percent of the drug is absorbed into the bloodstream with nasal spray usage.
- Metabolism of the absorbed drug (how the body breaks down the drug) does not occur.
- The elimination of the drug (how the body gets rid of it) is accomplished by the kidneys and the intestines. Of the small amount found in the bloodstream, about half enters the bile and is eliminated by the intestines. The other half is found in the urine unchanged.
- The half-life of the drug (the amount of time it takes the body to remove half of the drug still circulating in the bloodstream) is about one to two hours.

Other Information

Since this drug is marketed as a nasal spray, the precautions associated with these OTC products should be followed (see pages 96-98).

Breast-feeding

No thorough studies on breast-feeding and this drug have been reported. However, the absorption of cromolyn sodium from the intestines is only one percent. Therefore, if this drug is ever found in breast milk, the amount absorbed from the baby's intestines would be so small that no effect would be seen. Therefore, it is probably safe to use cromolyn sodium at the recommended dose and frequency while breast-feeding.

15. Nighttime Sleep-Aids

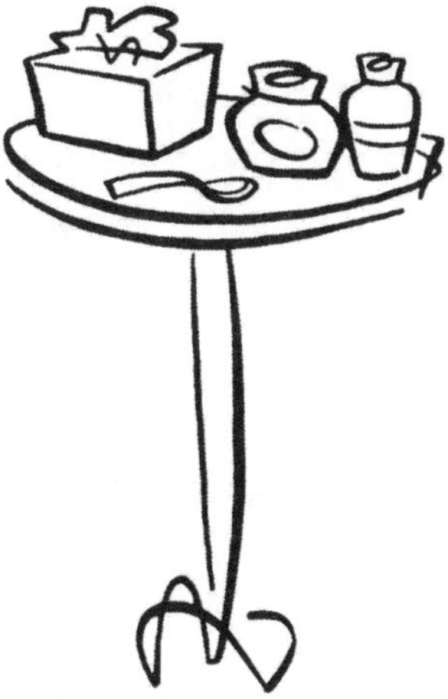

Sleep is a period of rest for the body and mind during which consciousness is partially or completely inactive. The inability to sleep is called **insomnia**. You may wonder why this topic is covered in a book about OTC cold remedies. The answer lies with the medications that are currently available over-the-counter as nighttime sleep-aids. These drugs are antihistamines and were covered in detail in Chapter 8.

What Is Normal?

A common misconception is that eight hours of sleep at night constitutes a good night's rest and is the normal amount needed. Actually, defining normal sleep time is probably not possible because what is normal for one person may not be normal for the next.

One of the best ways to determine whether a person is obtaining an adequate amount of sleep time is to analyze his or her daytime. If a person's daytime mood, function, and wakefulness are not impaired, then a satisfactory amount of sleep has probably occurred. Some people just need less sleep than others.

Because it is difficult to define normal sleep time, insomnia is also difficult to characterize. Insomnia is often categorized into short-term or transient (less than three to four weeks) versus long-term or chronic (more than three to four weeks).

The Endless List

The list of potential causes for insomnia is endless. However, the inciting factors can usually be grouped into a few categories which are emotional stress (such as family, work, school), physical stress, illness, drugs (caffeine and others), poor sleep habits, and age.

Most of us, at some time, have had difficulty falling asleep prior to a big event, such as a test, speech, or presentation. This is normal. However, some emotional stresses can be long term, especially if they are family or job related.

Regular exercise usually promotes better sleep. However, if a person is physically stressed beyond his or her limits or they develop an illness, normal continuous restful sleep may be difficult to achieve. This type of insomnia usually improves when the physical stress and/or illness has passed.

All of us should know that certain drugs like caffeine and related chemicals promote wakefulness. These substances may be found in coffee, tea, certain sodas, and chocolate. Another common drug group is the over-the-counter decongestants.

Insomnia may also be induced by many prescription medications and drugs that are abused (cocaine and amphetamines). Alcohol is a drug that most people associate with promoting sleep. However, sleep after moderate to heavy alcohol consumption is usually not continuous and restful. In many cases, the brain cannot maintain sleep, and the person will wake up several times during the night.

For many of us, the older we get, the less sleep we need. Although several explanations for this phenomenon have been suggested, napping during the day may be at the top of the list. If a person naps during the day, he or she will usually need less sleep at night. On the other hand, the more active a person is during the day, the more time will be spent in sleeping at night.

Finally, many people claim to have insomnia when in fact, they have poor sleep habits. These individuals may sleep with a light on or with a television or radio playing. Although sleeping with an ongoing outside stimulus is possible, eventually the brain will take notice causing the person to wake up, only to fall asleep again. This sleep is not continuous and may not be restful. Therefore, when sleeping, try to have as little outside interference as possible.

Pregnancy And Insomnia

Some women may experience insomnia during pregnancy. The list of potential causes can include the entire discussion above. In addition, tremendous changes occur in a woman's body when she is pregnant. These include changes in hormonal patterns, physiology, metabolism, physical stress (not relieved until delivery), and emotional stress (continues into motherhood). Emotional stress during pregnancy often involves the excitement and uncertainty of what is to come. All of these feelings are normal but treatment can be difficult.

Have You Ever Noticed?

Have you ever noticed that certain things, such as pain, become more intense at night? In reality, pain does not increase at night but rather is more focused. During the day, the brain analyzes a tremendous amount of simultaneous input by comprehending light and dark, colors, noises, sensations, smells, pains, and many other things all at the same time. At night, however, the majority of these stimuli greatly decrease. If something on the body is sore, the brain tends to focus on the problem and, therefore, it seems more intense.

This concept is also true for "the things that need to get done." Many of us (myself included) will go to bed and think about all the things we need to accomplish in the next day or two. This mental exercise can keep us awake, at which point we tell ourselves "I have too much to do tomorrow, so I need to fall asleep!" Unfortunately, this can sometimes make it even more difficult to fall asleep by causing anxiety (over not falling asleep). In such situations, doing something else (like reading) may help to divert the thinking process to another topic until sleepiness develops. In addition, medications can occasionally be used for these periodic occurrences.

The over-the-counter medications for treating insomnia are **only for temporary use** of occasional nighttime sleep difficulties. They are not meant for long-time usage. If you are pregnant and having difficulty sleeping at night (to the point where it affects your functioning the next day), talk with your healthcare provider before you seek drug treatment.

Another Job Made Easy

The FDA has again made my job easy in the category of nighttime sleep-aids. Several years ago, many different medications were available over-the-counter. Now only two remain. Prior to the FDA's review, there were several antihistamine drugs, bromides, and a few anticholinergic medications. The bromide drugs and anticholinergic medications were not approved because they were found to be ineffective at the doses seen in OTC products. To become effective, higher doses would be needed, reaching a level that was no longer considered safe over-the-counter.

Likewise, several antihistamine drugs were available; however, the list was decreased to two. These are **diphenhydramine** and **doxylamine**, and both were discussed in Chapter 8, Antihistamines. Some of the FDA recommended wording for the nighttime sleep-aids is: relief of occasional sleeplessness, helps you fall asleep, or reduces time to falling asleep.

Diphenhydramine

Diphenhydramine (di-fen-HI-dra-meen) is one of the available OTC ingredients that may be found in nighttime sleep-aids. This drug was discussed in detail on pages 149-153. The **Warnings**, **Drug Interactions**, and **Side Effects** sections should also be read (pages 140-143). Common brand name (trade name) medications that contain this ingredient are Nytol and Sominex. However, remember that the active ingredients in a brand name product can change over time. Therefore, you still need to read the labels.

This medication is recommended for use only once a night. Also, you should not take this drug concurrently with alcohol, sedatives, tranquilizers, or other drugs that cause drowsiness. While taking this medicine, if the insomnia continues for more than one to two weeks, you should talk with your healthcare provider.

Doxylamine

Doxylamine (dox-ILL-am-meen) is the other available OTC ingredient that may be found in nighttime sleep-aids. This drug was discussed in detail on pages 153-156. The **Warnings**, **Drug Interactions**, and **Side Effects** sections should also be read (pages 140-143). A common brand name (trade name) medication that contains this ingredient is Unisom. However, remember that the active ingredients in a brand name product can change over time. Therefore, you still need to read the labels.

This medication is recommended for use only once a night. Also, you should not take this drug concurrently with alcohol, sedatives, tranquilizers, or other drugs that cause drowsiness. While taking this medicine, if the insomnia continues for more than one to two weeks, you should talk with your healthcare provider.

16. Drug Reference & Dosage Equivalency Guide

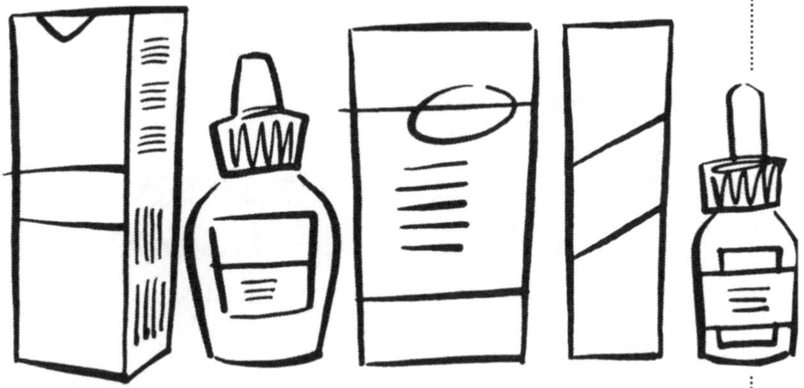

Drug ingredients, their classifications, and where they may be found in this book are listed below. These drugs are mainly found in over-the-counter cold remedies, medicines for treating sore throats, eye medications, drugs for asthma and respiratory allergies, and nighttime sleep-aids. In addition, a few of the listed drugs may no longer be found in over-the-counter medications but might be contained in products called **natural remedies** (homeopathic medicines) that can still be purchased over-the-counter. The ingredients in these natural remedies are also very important for pregnant women to know about.

On page 258, you will find a handy **Dosage Equivalency Guide** that can be used to make comparisons between cubic centimeters (cc), milliliters (ml), and teaspoons (tsp). This can help a person determine how much medicine to take based on what is recommended by a healthcare provider or printed on a package label.

PLEASE remember, **over-the-counter medicines are drugs** and if you are pregnant, they might affect your pregnancy. If you decide to use an over-the-counter drug during your pregnancy, please read about the active ingredients discussed in this book, and please talk with your healthcare provider before using the medication.

Active Ingredients Discussed In This Book

Other Ingredients Mentioned

14. The belladonna drugs may still be found in some **natural remedies** and some of the names for these ingredients are listed below (see pages 209-212).

Atropa belladonna
Atropine
Belladonna extract
Datura stramonium
Deadly nightshade
Devil's apple
Homatropine
Hyoscine
Hyoscyamine
Hyoscyamus niger
Jamestown weed
Jimson weed
Methscopolamine
Scopolamine
Scopolia carniolica
Stink weed
Thorn-apple
Tincture of belladonna

Dosage Equivalency Guide

A cubic centimeter or cc, is the same as a milliliter or ml, and it takes five of either to equal a teaspoon or tsp.

¼ teaspoon	=	1.25 cc or 1.25 ml
½ teaspoon	=	2.5 cc or 2.5 ml
¾ teaspoon	=	3.75 cc or 3.75 ml
1 teaspoon	=	5 cc or 5 ml
2 teaspoons	=	10 cc or 10 ml
1 tablespoon	=	15 cc or 15 ml (1 tablespoon = 3 teaspoons)
1 ounce	=	30 cc or 30 ml (1 ounce = 2 tablespoons = 6 teaspoons)
1 pint	=	16 ounces (or about 480 cc)

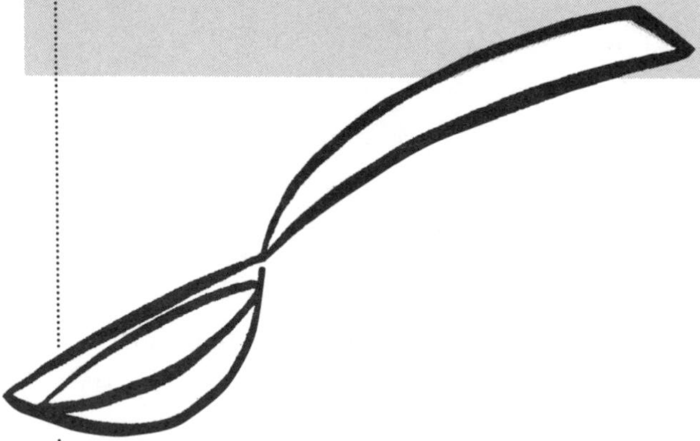

Appendix

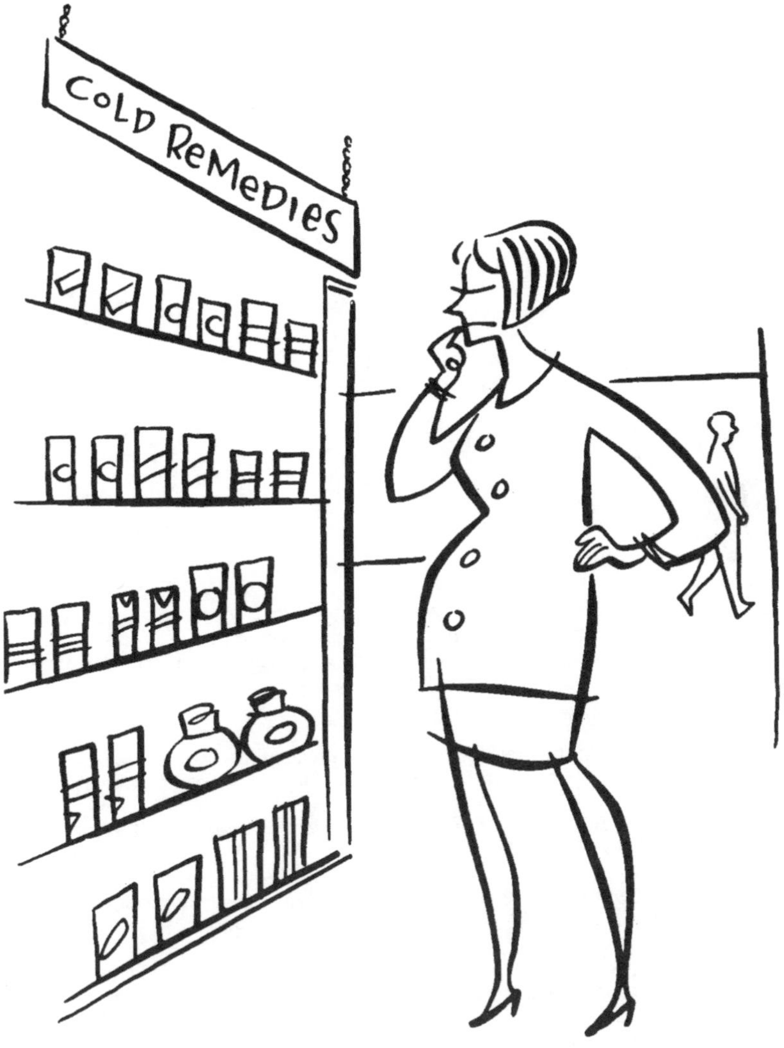

Table 1: The number of patients reported who had first trimester exposures to decongestant-type drugs (including asthma and eye medications) from three large random pregnant populations.

Active Ingredient	CPP	MMSS	GHCPS	Total
1. Oxymetazoline	2		255*	257*
2. Xylometazoline	8		461	469
3. Naphazoline	20			20
4. Propylhexedrine	5			5
5. Phenylephrine	1,249		401*	1,650*
6. Pseudoephedrine	39	940	1,530	2,509
7. Phenylpropanolamine	726		354*	1,080*
8. Levmetamfetamine ** (L-desoxyephedrine)	671			671
9. Epinephrine (asthma)	189	35		224
10. Ephedrine (asthma)	373	96		469
11. Tetrahydrozoline (eye only)	3			3

* The data from the GHCPS are from two publications and, therefore, the numbers for the active ingredients were combined. In the first report, a range of usage (of 100 to 199 women) was listed for a few of the medications. Thus, to be conservative, only a minimum value of 100 was added to the number of patients reported in the second publication.

** The numbers listed in the table for this active ingredient are actually for amphetamine drugs in general and not specifically for levmetamfetamine.

CPP The CPP is the Collaborative Perinatal Project that evaluated 50,282 pregnancies from 1959 through 1965.

MMSS The MMSS is the Michigan Medicaid Surveillance Study that evaluated 333,440 pregnancies from 1980 through 1983 and from 1985 to mid-1992.

GHCPS The GHCPS is the Group Health Cooperative of Puget Sound, Seattle, Washington that evaluated 13,346 pregnancies from mid-1977 to mid-1982.

These three studies are discussed in detail on pages 60-62.

Table 2: The number of patients reported who had first trimester exposures to the antihistamine drugs from three large random pregnant populations.

Active Ingredient	CPP	MMSS	GHCPS	Total
1. Diphenhydramine	595	2,898	631	4,124
2. Doxylamine	1,169	5,995	3,834	10,998
3. Clemastine		1,831		1,831
4. Chlorpheniramine	1,070	1,154	357*	2,581*
5. Dexchlorpheniramine		1,080		1,080
6. Brompheniramine	65	859	272*	1,196*
7. Dexbrompheniramine	14	471		485
8. Pheniramine	831			831
9. Triprolidine	16	910	628	1,554
10. Pyrilamine	121			121
11. Chlorcyclizine	13			13
12. Phenindamine	12			12
13. Thonzylamine	148			148

* The data from the GHCPS are from two publications and, therefore, the numbers for the active ingredients were combined. In the first report, a range of usage (of 100 to 199 women) was listed for a few of the medications. Thus, to be conservative, only a minimum value of 100 was added to the number of patients reported in the second publication.

CPP The CPP is the Collaborative Perinatal Project that evaluated 50,282 pregnancies from 1959 through 1965.

MMSS The MMSS is the Michigan Medicaid Surveillance Study that evaluated 333,440 pregnancies from 1980 through 1983 and from 1985 to mid-1992.

GHCPS The GHCPS is the Group Health Cooperative of Puget Sound, Seattle, Washington that evaluated 13,346 pregnancies from mid-1977 to mid-1982.

These three studies are discussed in detail on pages 60-62.

Table 3: The number of patients reported who had first trimester exposures to cough suppressants and expectorants from three large random pregnant populations.

Active Ingredient	CPP	MMSS	GHCPS	Total
Cough Suppressants				
1. Dextromethorphan	300		59	359
2. Codeine	563	13,020	1,204*	14,787*
3. Diphenhydramine	595	2,898	631	4,124
4. Chlophedianol	1			1
5. Camphor	168			168
6. Menthol				0
Expectorants				
1. Guaifenesin	197	141	740*	1,078*

* The data from the GHCPS are from two publications and, therefore, the numbers for the active ingredients were combined. In the first report, a range of usage (of 100 to 199 women) was listed for a few of the medications. Thus, to be conservative, only a minimum value of 100 was added to the number of patients reported in the second publication.

CPP The CPP is the Collaborative Perinatal Project that evaluated 50,282 pregnancies from 1959 through 1965.

MMSS The MMSS is the Michigan Medicaid Surveillance Study that evaluated 333,440 pregnancies from 1980 through 1983 and from 1985 to mid-1992.

GHCPS The GHCPS is the Group Health Cooperative of Puget Sound, Seattle, Washington that evaluated 13,346 pregnancies from mid-1977 to mid-1982.

These three studies are discussed in detail on pages 60-62.

Table 4: The effects of alpha and beta drugs on various parts of the body.

Alpha Drugs

Part of the Body	Effect of the Alpha Drug
Heart	Causes it to beat harder and faster (heart rate increases)
Blood Vessels - including blood vessels to the uterus	Causes them to constrict (increases blood pressure and may decrease the amount of blood that goes to an area)
Pancreas	Decreases release of insulin* (may increase blood sugar)
Liver	Breaks down stored-up sugar (may increase blood sugar)
Intestines	Relaxes the muscles of the intestines
Uterus	Could cause the muscles to contract (may promote contractions)

* Insulin is the hormone that helps to regulate blood sugar.

Beta Drugs

Part of the Body	Effect of the Beta Drug
Heart (beta-1)	Causes it to beat harder and faster (heart rate increases)
Blood Vessels - including blood vessels to the uterus (beta-2)	Causes them to relax (may decrease blood pressure)
Lungs (beta-2)	Causes muscles in the lungs to relax (may allow a person to breathe easier)
Liver (beta-2)	Breaks down stored-up sugar (may increase blood sugar)
Uterus (beta-2)	Causes the muscles to relax (may decrease or stop contractions)

Most beta drugs have both beta-1 and beta-2 activity. Some specific medications may be more active in one area over the other.

Table 5: **The effects of the substance called histamine on various parts of the body.**

Part of the Body	The Effect of Histamine
Lungs	Causes muscles in the lungs to constrict (makes it more difficult for a person to breathe)
Blood Vessel Muscles	May cause them to relax (may lower blood pressure)
Nerves	Irritates nerve endings (may cause itching)
Tissue and Blood Vessels	Causes them to be leaky (may cause swelling and irritation)
Intestinal Muscles	Causes them to contract (may cause cramping)
Stomach	Increases the release of stomach acid (may cause heartburn, stomachaches, or promote/irritate ulcers)

Antihistamine drugs try to block some of the above-listed effects. However, they do not block the release of histamine.

Bibliography

Over 500 resources were used in the preparation of this work, therefore, only selected references are listed below. The first items (Nos. 1, 2, and 3) correspond to the three major studies described in Chapter 4 and are referred to by superior numbers throughout the text.

1. Heinonen O.P., Slone D., and Shapiro S. *Birth Defects and Drugs in Pregnancy*, Boston: John Wright, PSG Inc., 1983.

2. Rosa F., and Baum C. "Medicaid Surveillance of Drugs in Pregnancy and Birth Defects." Rockville, Maryland: U.S. Food And Drug Administration, Freedom of Information, 1995.

3. Jick H., Holmes L.B., Hunter J.R., Madsen S., and Stergachis A."First-trimester Drug Use and Congential Disorders." *Journal of the American Medical Association*: **246**: 343-346, 1981. (and) Aselton P., Jick H., Milunsky A., Hunter J.R., and Stergachis A."First-trimester Drug Use and Congenital Disorders." *Obstetrics and Gynecology*: **65**: 451-455, 1985.

American Academy of Pediatrics, Committee on Drugs. "The Transfer of Drugs and Other Chemicals Into Human Milk." *Pediatrics*: **93**: 137-150, 1994.

Baxi L.V., Gindoff P.R., Pregenzer G.J., and Parras M.K. "Fetal Heart Rate Changes Following Maternal Administration of a Nasal Decongestant." *American Journal of Obstetrics and Gynecology*: **153**: 799-800, 1985.

Brocklebank J.C., Ray W.A., Federspiel C.F., and Schaffner W. "Drug Prescribing During Pregnancy. A Controlled Study of Tennessee Medicaid Recipients." *American Journal of Obstetrics and Gynecology*: **132**: 235-244, 1978.

Code of Federal Regulations 21, Parts 300 to 499, U.S. Food and Drug Administration. Published by the Office of the Federal Register, National Archives and Records Administration. Washington, D.C. 1998.

Consumer Healthcare Products Association - List of Ingredients and Dosages Transferred from Rx-to-OTC Status (or New Over-The-Counter Approvals) by the FDA from 1975 through April 1999.

Cottle M.K.W., Van Petten G.R., and Van Muyden P. "Effects of Phenylephrine and Sodium Salicylate on Maternal and Fetal Cardiovascular Indices and Blood Oxygenation in Sheep." *American Journal of Obstetrics and Gynecology*: **143**: 170-176, 1982.

Council on Scientific Affairs - American Medical Association. "Saccharin: Review of Safety Issues." *Journal of the American Medical Association*: **254**: 2622-2624, 1985.

Doering P.L., and Stewart R.B. "The Extent and Character of Drug Consumption During Pregnancy." *Journal of the American Medical Association*: **239**: 843-846, 1978.

Drug Monographs from the U.S. Food and Drug Administration on Over-The-Counter Ingredients. Final Rulings: Cough/Cold-Nasal Decongestant , Cough/Cold-Antihistamine, Cough/Cold-Antitussive, Cough/Cold-Expectorant, Cough/Cold-Anticholinergic, Cough/Cold-Bronchodilator, Daytime Sedatives, and Nighttime Sleep-aid, Federal Register - CFR 21. Washington, D.C. Various publications from 1979 through 1997.

Hardman J.G., Limbird L.E., Molinoff P.B., Ruddon R.W., Gilman A.G., Eds. Goodman and Gilman's - *The Pharmacological Basis of Therapeutics*, 9th Edition. New York: McGraw-Hill Publishing Co. Inc., 1996.

Holmes L.B. "Teratogen Update: Bendectin." *Teratology*: **27**: 277-281, 1983.

Micromedix DrugDex® Pharmaceutical Computer Program. Micromedix, Inc. Colorado: 1998.

Milkovich L., and van den Berg B.J. "Effects of Antenatal Exposure to Anorectic Drugs." *American Journal of Obstetrics and Gynecology*: **129**: 637-642, 1977.

O'Brien T.E. "Excretion of Drugs In Human Milk." *American Journal of Hospital Pharmacy*: **31**: 844-854, 1974.

Physicians' Desk Reference (PDR). New Jersey: Medical Economics Publishing, selected editions from 1949 through 1999.

Physicians' Desk Reference for Nonprescription Drugs and Dietary Supplements. New Jersey: Medical Economics Publishing, selected editions from 1980 through 1999.

Physicians Desk Reference Guide to Drug Interaction, Side Effects, Indications, Contraindications. New Jersey: Medical Economics Publishing, 1997.

Piper J.M., Baum C., and Kennedy D.L. "Prescription Drug Use Before and During Pregnancy in a Medicaid Population." *American Journal of Obstetrics and Gynecology*: **157**: 148-156, 1987.

Rayburn W.F., Anderson J.C., Smith C.V., Appel L.L., and Davis S.A. "Uterine and Fetal Doppler Flow Changes From a Single Dose of a Long-Acting Intranasal Decongestant." *Obstetrics and Gynecology*: **76**: 180-182, 1990.

Stegink L.D. "The Aspartame Story: A Model for the Clinical Testing of a Food Additive." *American Journal of Clinical Nutrition*: **46**: 204-215, 1987.

Wilson J. "Use of Sodium Cromoglycate During Pregnancy: Results on 296 Asthmatic Women." *Acta Therapeutica*: **8** (supplement): 45-51, 1982.

Wright R.G., Shnider S.M., Levinson G., Rolbin S.H. and Parer J.T. "The Effect of Maternal Administration of Ephedrine on Fetal Heart Rate Variability." *Obstetrics and Gynecology*: **57**: 734-738, 1981.

Index

a

b

e-f

g-h

i-j-k

q-r-s

t-z